ANTONOV

ANTONOV
My Story
Roumen Antonov

READ BOOKS

WARNING

To experiment with the medication 'M' described herein can be dangerous to health and life if done without professional guidance and control. The author warns all against attempting any of the procedures described.

First published in Bulgaria 1998 by Pygmalion Press, Plovdiv

This revised English edition published in 1999 by

ISBN 0 9534186-0-X

The right of Roumen Antonov to be identified as the author of this work has been asserted by him in accordance with Sections 77 and 78 of the Copyright, Designs and Patents Act 1988.

Copyright © Roumen Antonov 1999

All rights reserved. No part of this publication may be reproduced, stored in or introduced into a retrieval system, or transmitted, in any form, or by any means (electronic, mechanical, photocopying, recording or otherwise) without the prior written permission of the Publisher. Any person who does any unauthorized act in relation to this publication may be liable to criminal prosecution and civil claims for damages.

British Library Cataloguing in Publication Data.

A catalogue record for this book is available from the British Library.

Edited by Robin Read
Design and layout by Matthew Yorke
Printed and bound in Great Britain by
Biddles Ltd, Guildford, Surrey

To the memory of my grandmother Stoena
and mother Evgenya.

Their enduring spirit and constant belief in me has
inspired and sustained my work through all adversity

ACKNOWLEDGEMENTS

I have received help from a great many people during the preparation of this book. I should like to thank my business partners Mike Emmerson and Cees Minnaar for their unfailing support. I am also particularly grateful to Rusi Dundakov, Roxanne Summers, Pierrot Meyer, Marie-France Hugot, Diana Brandsema, my translator Anna Moskova and editor Robin Read.

Contents

List of Illustrations

	Preface	9
1	Family and Childhood	11
2	Those long school years	23
3	Military Service	39
4	What will I be when I grow up?	47
5	Profession and Hobby	57
6	Wandering in a Maze	67
7	The Four-Stroke engine	77
8	Vocation: Bastard	85
9	The Unattainable Calm	95
10	Candida Albicans	103
11	Dancing with the Devil	115
12	Wiesbaden	127
13	The Price of Freedom	137
14	The Antonov Automatic Gearbox	145
15	Drawing to an End	155
16	Epilogue	161
	Appendix: Bulgaria - the Roots	163
	Index	174

List of Illustrations

Between pages 32 and 33
1. Grandmother's house in the village of Dolni Lozen
2. Grandmother Stoena and her sister in Shopp costume
3. Grandmother's family in the late Twenties
4. Grandmother and Mother at the end of the Thirties
5. My father Anton in the late Thirties
6. Mother and I in Spring 1944
7. The little street urchin of 1946
8. A Horch 853
9. My brother Evgeni and I in the late Forties
10. Mother with my brother Evgeni and me

Between pages 64 and 65
11. Vlady Udrev with Father on the DKW 125
12. Adriana, my brother and Rosalina
13. With Bobby in the City Garden
14. Shortly before my arrest in 1961
15. Army Days
16. Grandmother visited me at the garrison
17. The Family Antonov in 1964
18. Vera and I passing the Alexander Nevski cathedral
19. Rositsa
20. Student days with the Renault 8

Between pages 96 and 97
21. Reflecting on problems
22. My son Viktor
23. Movie art director in 1973
24. Aged twenty-nine
25. My marriage to Galya
26. Viktor and I in the Swinging Seventies
27. In 1979 I began my experiments
28. In 1986 I considered marriage
29. Roxanne

Between pages 128 and 129
30. At work in my attic
31. A scale model of my coupé
32. Edith and I
33. Starting the motor of the model car
34. My model at rest
35. Pierrot and his wife trail away the Peugeot 305
36. The Antonov automatic transmission
37. With Dan Wysenbeek
38. In front of the workshop
39. In a Peugeot 205
40. Jean-Claude completing assembly
41. I was granted French citizenship in Lorraine
42. In Tokyo, 1993
43. At the Mortefontaine test track
44. Testing the prototype of my engine
45. Writing *My Story* at home
46. Fungal blastospores
47. Fungal micellae

Preface

This book is my life story to date; the adventure of a 'loner' who succeeded in escaping from one side of the Iron Curtain to successfully begin a new life and introduce a major invention in the automotive industry.

In 1988 after many futile attempts to escape from the communist regime in the country of my birth, Bulgaria, I finally managed to reach Paris. Then quite unexpectedly, the communist regime in Sofia was toppled a year and a half later.

When I reached the West I was forty-four, a newly-arrived emigrant unable to speak French and without money and friends. My life in Bulgaria had been completely ruined following my refusal to engage in work on behalf of the secret institutions of the Bulgarian State Security, a branch of the KGB.

In 1979 I began work on a biological experiment that could be of the greatest importance to the course of medicine. At the time however it was impossible for me to publish the results of my work despite enormous efforts to do so. I then discovered nine years later that it was just as impossible for a refugee to publish anything on a new medical discovery in the West.

As I had also developed a couple of engineering inventions I thought that it might be easier to launch one of them, my automatic gearbox, in the car industry. But how could I have possibly imagined that as a penniless refugee such an enterprise could have any chance at all of success?

As I look back on my experiences my optimism at that time seems totally illogical but nevertheless the project turned out well and here I find myself writing this story just as I knew I would. Without the clear success that it has been my good fortune to achieve, the story would have seemed so improbable that I cannot imagine that anyone would have believed it.

Roumen Antonov
Paris

Chapter One
Family and Childhood

No member of my family played a greater role in my life than my maternal grandmother Stoena. She was the most energetic person I have ever known.

In small villages at the foot of the mountains rising above Sofia live the *Shopps*, possibly the most unusual among Bulgarian people. Stubbornness is without question their most distinctive feature and we may assume that this quality resulted from a continuing need for self-preservation and survival. The famed obstinacy and pig-headedness of the Shopps has given rise to many jokes about their suspicion of everything lying beyond their village boundary.

My grandmother was born in one of the Shopp villages, Dolni Lozen, at the beginning of this century. Dolni Lozen is situated a mere 20km from the centre of Sofia but at that time seemed totally isolated from the rest of the world. In the upper part of the village at the foot of the mountain lived the Gyokov family. There was no aristocracy or even bourgeoisie to create class distinctions in Bulgarian villages and everyone worked together ploughing and hoeing or herding sheep. So it was their distinctive stubbornness that marked out the renowned Gyokov family among their fellow villagers.

This was the family into which my grandmother was born and just like everyone else was sent to care for a flock of sheep rather than to study at school. She grew up a large-framed, sturdy young woman with great strength - highly praised qualities among the Shopps. The Gyokov family's doggedness permeated her character and led her to fall in love and marry a man from another village - an act of reckless folly strongly opposed and instantly rejected by the unthinkingly conservative Shopp villagers.

My grandfather Svetoslav Ignatov (*Slavcho*) was born in another Shopp village, Lesnovo. He was a man of great serenity and patience and never once raised his voice in my presence. When the robust young bride came to live with her husband's parents the traditional animosity between mother-in-law and daughter-in-law, especially those from differing villages, quickly developed to an alarming degree. Docility was not in Grandmother's nature and it was not surprising that she soon packed her belongings and with my grandfather and their newborn baby, my mother Evgenya, departed for Sofia.

The arrival of yet another Shopp family in the capital during the 1920s was merely another insignificant example of Bulgaria's increasing march towards civilisation. Here was a family in a horse-drawn cart loaded with a few rugs and other meagre possessions, directed by my grandmother's energy and determination towards a strange new world; one into which I too, would later be born. In the meantime my grandmother planned to sail the family ship on an unswerving course towards prosperity.

In the Twenties Sofia could offer few opportunities to a couple of illiterate peasants seeking employment. Anything - even the dirtiest and lowest paid work - must have been warmly welcomed by my grandparents. They began their new life in great poverty on the bottom rung of the ladder with my grandmother working as a servant and my grandfather as a building labourer.

However, in less than twenty years the family had undergone a profound change. By now my grandmother had two daughters and was a lady of leisure. In her spacious apartment in the centre of Sofia at the junction of two of the most beautiful boulevards and facing the Czar's palace, she enjoyed all the privileges of middle class life - modern furniture, a lift, telephone and radio. All this was cared for by a servant girl. My grandmother dressed in the latest Paris fashions; wearing elegant clothes made by a dressmaker who came to the house for fittings. She visited the most expensive restaurants in Sofia and each summer spent a month at the luxurious Black Sea resort of Varna in the company of her two daughters, whose lives were now suffused with the romance of *Gone With The Wind*, then sweeping the world.

So these two illiterate peasants had been able to work their way up as a result of their hard work and ability to adapt to change. My grandmother was the ambitious architect of that progress; it was she who carefully chose the new addresses, roles and acquaintances. My grandfather was a clever, hard-working man but he was also quiet and good-natured and only too happy to follow his energetic wife's lead in developing the family's strategy for the future. After a series of odd jobs he finally achieved success by establishing a small business making leather coats, with a workshop where he could apply his skills to the craft. It was thanks to his success that Grandmother Stoena, born and raised in a primitive isolated village, could now aspire to the position of a lady in a modern city. Nevertheless, this would not have been achieved without Stoena's will, energetic application and courage.

Grandmother was not a cultured woman. She was almost illiterate and had the greatest difficulty in reading and writing. Her childhood had been spent in a house at the very end of the village with the Lozen mountain rising beyond the garden fence. To ward off the evil spirits that lurked in the hills and came down at night and along the valley to the very gates of the houses, people could only resort to prayer and the protection of the cross. It was unquestioning faith that compensated for the illiteracy of Grandmother and countless generations of Bulgarians. As they were unable to read the Bible, religion was practised by means of fables and rites coupled with passionate worship and devotion to individual saints. Against the overwhelming forces of darkness and witchcraft my grandmother sought the protection of Saint Mennas; a choice that henceforth saved her from any form of moral or inner conflict.

St Mennas gave Grandmother the strongest feeling of self-righteousness throughout her life and defended her against all intellectual or spiritual interference. I assume that this was probably why my grandmother never appeared to suffer from her lack of education. For example, throughout her life she believed that the earth was flat. No arguments, however scientific, from the time of Columbus up to modern satellites, including hard evidence in the form of several transatlantic flights to the United States, could convince her that she was wrong and she pitied others for their ignorance of the truth. As far as education was concerned she was convinced that if her father had sent her to school instead of to shepherd sheep, she would have become a government minister at least.

Grandmother had a strong personality and her character was such that she would undoubtedly have made a leader of some kind. Her presence and self-confidence was boundless but her iron will was somewhat excessive, as both her daughters frequently experienced.

My mother Evgenya had my grandfather's calm disposition. She could remember her grandfather Ignat, a tall and handsome man whose good looks she had inherited. Her

Family and Childhood

beauty gave her the harmony, natural poise and grace of children adored at an early age and although she was a romantic schoolgirl and a rather undistinguished student she became the object of passionate longing to many admirers; some of whom remained faithful friends throughout her life.

Conflict was inevitable between Grandmother and Mother. Totally bereft of all romance, my grandmother's essentially practical mind regarded Mother's natural beauty as a God-given asset to be controlled and exploited in exchange for the social status and material wealth of a good marriage. Under the influence of the sentimental fiction of the 1930s, my romantic mother suffered greatly at the hands of her tyrannical parent. Nevertheless, love triumphed.

My father Anton was a young army lieutenant when he won Mother's heart shortly before the Second World War. Grandmother Stoena would naturally have to approve the relationship before it could result in marriage. Unfortunately for the devoted couple, Grandmother had made enquiries about the suitor Anton and had rejected him out of hand.

Father was born in Vidin, a beautiful old town in north west Bulgaria on the western bank of the Danube. My grandfather Otto was a bank manager with a large estate, a passion for hunting and a fine motorcar. Grandmother Borislava was a graduate of the Academy of Fine Arts. Sadly, my grandfather Otto died young and his widow had to sell everything to pay for the education of their four children. Nevertheless, because the family's property was converted into his education, my father's performance at the high school must have been a good investment. As the best student he was immediately admitted to the military school and on graduation was able to embark on a distinguished army career. My father had also achieved good results in science and although that was not essential for success, it marked him out among his fellows.

Soon after commissioning as an officer he was stationed in Sofia where with his fellow subalterns he thoroughly enjoyed the pleasures of life in his fine uniform and sword; cutting a dash in the restaurants and casinos of the prewar capital. But Father, like many of these other young officers, had very little beyond his uniform, sword and modest army pay.

It was this that concerned my grandmother. She had an inner instinct which rejected my father as a fellow being, but fundamentally it was his lack of wealth that prevented him from meeting her approval as a future son-in-law.

In the first months of the war, conflict of a similar nature developed between Grandmother and Mother. Before the tide of war which would soon disrupt the lives of so many, the famous Shopp stubbornness now created a melodrama of passionate love. Grandmother was determined to put an end to my parents' romance and to introduce another, more eligible suitor by force if necessary. The situation was complicated by the fact that Grandmother's nominee was also an army officer, in love with Mother but most important of all, well-to-do. With characteristic resolution, Grandmother attempted to impose her will by intimidation, threats and restrictions; often in the presence of my horrified father. A mere nineteen year-old girl, Mother was unable to resist and eventually was forced to give way.

As always in youthful affairs of the heart, passions ran high. Separated by my tyrannical grandmother, the two lovers yearned for each other yet more, but in my mother's blood the Shopp stubbornness overruled all other emotions. While my distraught father took comfort in the bottle when his Beloved's engagement to another man was announced, my mother relentlessly schemed to undermine my domineering grandmother. At great risk and only a few days after her engagement to my father's dreaded rival she sent the pining

Anton a letter promising unswerving devotion, and the two lovers met secretly to plan victory over my grandmother.

Grandmother was easily flattered and was lured out of town by an invitation to take lunch with the rejected suitor. During this outing Mother was supposed to behave like a polite but indifferent friend towards her former admirer. My father hired a car and drove mother and daughter to Boyana, a small village at the foot of the Vitosha mountain that rises behind Sofia. After lunch at the famous Chepishev restaurant, the party visited one of Bulgaria's oldest shrines, the Boyana Church, built in the thirteenth century and housing the frescos of Theodor and Desislava the great medieval king and his consort. Before the most ancient surviving image of true Bulgarians, Father took out his sword, aimed it at Grandmother and forced her to kneel before the icon of the Virgin Mary to swear in the saint's name that she would give him her daughter's hand.

This time St Mennas failed to come to the assistance of Grandmother and she dared not refuse. However her dislike of my father was henceforth transformed into deep and enduring hatred.

Mother fully understood Grandmother's character and knew that she would keep her word. My mother was very religious too, but more in the tradition of the Bible and the Orthodox faith. Each morning and evening she prayed and nothing could distract her at those times. I have never seen anyone so truly religious, and her inner harmony and peace, nourished by faith, gave her deep happiness.

Aided by the involvement of so many important saints, my parents finally and inevitably were married at St Cyriaca's Church where twenty years earlier a bomb hurled by a Communist had narrowly missed the Czar but killed many bystanders.

My brother Lyuben was born a year before me. When only a month old, he caught severe pneumonia and died. Grandmother had learned from a fortune teller that the omens were bad from the beginning of his unfortunate life.

The war was beginning to affect Bulgaria deeply. A period of acute shortages was accompanied by general poverty; the Czar died and the first Allied air raids terrified the population in Sofia. As an ally of Germany, Bulgaria was ordered by Hitler to send its army to occupy Macedonia. Father was stationed there and left Mother pregnant again, this time expecting me. During the autumn and winter of 1943 the bombing of Sofia intensified. Ivanka, Grandmother's servant girl, was the first to hear the drone of the approaching aircraft and apparently wet herself with fear. In the sky over the city a few desperate Bulgarian fighter pilots tried to attack the endless waves of Flying Fortresses. One of them, Spisarevski, finding himself out of ammunition, deliberately crashed his fighter into one of the American bombers. Whenever there was an air raid, Mother now heavily pregnant, went down to the shelter like everyone else. Soon the casualties from the air raids and the general destruction around them forced the family to leave Sofia and make their way to the small village of Malo Buchino in the mountains above the capital.

As she awaited my arrival, Mother sadly watched Sofia bombed and ruined before her eyes. The air raids became more frequent and heavier reaching a climax on 20 January 1944. Waves and waves of bombers virtually wiped out the city during the day and night - after darkness with the help of flares dropped by parachute. During her labour Mother remembered the terrifying sight of the city in flames punctuated by loud explosions as she lay fearfully in the tiny mountain village.

On the following day, during the morning of 21 January, I was born. That it was the day of Sofia's destruction from the air was not the only omen of my arrival in this world. I was

Family and Childhood

born in a caul which was considered a rare sign of good fortune and divine protection in the Shopps' tradition. In her absolute belief in Providence, Mother preserved my caul for years.

Nine months later, Russian troops entered the country and were received with flowers and enthusiasm by the local populace. The Bulgarian army stationed in German-occupied Macedonia was now turned against the *Wehrmacht* and Father was ordered to the Front. My parents had been separated for almost the entire duration of their marriage but Mother was now pregnant for the third time. `If the child is a boy give him your name, Evgeni, if it is a girl, name her Antonia after me' wrote Father in a passionate letter to his beloved wife who prayed fervently for his survival and a swift end to the war.

My brother Evgeni was born in March 1945, only six weeks before the war ended. Under orders from Moscow, the local Communist Party had taken over power in January and to many Bulgarians that quickly meant the end of their dreams and enthusiasm for a restored democracy. Decorated for bravery in action, my father soon had to swallow his disappointment because at the end of the war all Czarist officers were dismissed from the Bulgarian army. That was only a beginning however - to the new authorities a former Czarist officer in the family was good enough reason to throw out all of us from our spacious and luxurious apartment on Dondukov Boulevard.

Grandmother Stoena accepted this blow with stoicism. Everything she had carefully laboured to create was now destroyed. With two babes in arms and an unemployed husband, my Mother moved into a covered market where all our furniture and luggage was stored. In devastated post war Sofia severe repression and material shortages of every kind made the life of all dependant on the arbitrary behaviour of informers and minor bureaucrats. My grandmother set about fighting for her rights. She insisted that she was not a *bourgeoise* since she had come from a village, had worked as a servant and had taken part in strikes. That entitled her to rent two rooms in a heavily bomb-damaged apartment with the third room allotted to another family. The kitchen and bathroom were shared by both families.

My father found employment on a construction site. He enrolled as a student in the Polytechnic to study civil engineering. My grandfather's leather garment manufacturing company had been nationalised by the State but he could still earn enough from his craft to support the entire family. I can clearly remember the little sheepskin coats he made for my brother and me, with that same smell of tanned leather that always hung around.

My mother's younger sister Tanya had been overshadowed by my mother's beauty, poise and grace and remained in the background. In fact she was more adventurous and practical. Perhaps the subconscious competition had made her more ambitious and she never hesitated to take a difficult or unusual decision. While Mother still dreamed along in her romantic world, her sister Tanya decided to look elsewhere and, responding to Nazi propaganda enlisted for a job in Hitler's Germany. Disillusion was not long in arriving but not before love in the form of a German soldier brought relieving joy. Unfortunately Nazi race laws forbade the marriage of an Aryan to a Bulgarian girl and Hans was posted to the Eastern Front where he became a Russian prisoner of war, returning with both legs amputated to Germany twelve years later. Tanya gave birth to his son in Sofia at the same time that I was born but sadly this child died of pneumonia shortly thereafter. Thus far, good fortune had not smiled on Tanya. But she had the Shopp spirit and soon found new love in the form of Douglas, an airman in the Royal Air Force Mission in Sofia.

The British and American embassies in Sofia were treated with an increasing antipathy that soon turned into open hostility. Douglas and Tanya were married and left Sofia together with the Mission itself at the opening of the Cold War. Among my earliest memories is the smiling face of my Uncle Doug who had just drawn for me a Disney cartoon figure on a box lid. Vanished forever, he and Aunt Tanya became a myth in my life that continued to unroll like a film from my aunt's letters home and the numerous photographs she sent to us.

My father's sister fled the country too but she and her husband had defected at the height of Communist repression and were sentenced *in absentia*. They sank into oblivion in order not to give the authorities a pretext to persecute their relatives remaining in Bulgaria. Their three children, together with the five of my mother's sister Tanya, formed a colony of unknown to me cousins in the United States.

Among my earliest memories I recall the world seen from the window of the apartment in Graf Ignatiev Street where Grandmother had assembled her family. It was on the second floor of a building with a broken staircase and with kitchen and bathroom heavily damaged by American bombing. Below the windows trams rattled by. My grandparents, my brother and I slept in one room and the drawing room - separated by a glass door from the corridor - served as my parents' bedroom. Another family lived in the second room with their daughter and later, their son. My world was a tiny overcrowded place but I could spend hours sitting by the window watching the passers-by, the cars and trams in what was the busiest street of the capital.

To me the most exciting object of my childhood was the motorcar. Cars were magic animals to me and in my fantasy they became real creatures. Their presence amazed me; all their parts, surfaces and outlines were engraved forever in my memory. The cars that made this great impression upon me were rare and were mainly of German, Italian or American manufacture. My memories of some of these cars are still crystal-clear to this day. A godfather of my grandmother's family was Sokolov, a motor racing driver of the 1930s. He possessed a BMW 315; a two-seat convertible in blue and yellow that I still remember vividly.

Whenever I saw that car many years later I was always overcome by the same strong feelings of my childhood. The Sokolov family had maintained it in original condition and had driven it for more than thirty years. Sokolov himself and his small trophy room full of photographs, awards and cups are among the most enduring memories of my early years.

The feelings engendered by motorcars carried over to my toys. I did not have a single toy that represented the car I really cherished in my imagination. To have one was a dream that was forever unfulfilled. I still remember seeing a toy car displayed in a shop window. It was a white convertible with long elegant wings mounted on a chassis with all types of mechanism, in metal and with real rubber tyres. I was with my grandmother but she said that the toy was too expensive, clasped my hand and walked me away.

Among my earliest memories too are those of the chanting, singing crowds at the official parades organised by the Communist authorities. They wound along the streets for hours while my brother and I watched from a window the numerous placards painted in red and enormous portraits of mustachioed and bearded Communist leaders. The ugly, giant dummies with deformed faces personifying Uncle Sam carrying an atom bomb in his hand were spectacular; I remember distinctly a fat dummy of Tito brandishing a blood-stained hatchet above a slaughtered child in one hand while snatching dollars from Uncle Sam with the other. My brother was frightened, burst into tears and ran from the window. Later, and now inspired by the spectacle, my brother marched round the table in our crowded living room singing *Oh hero, hero, heroine*.

Family and Childhood

We would put a small chair in front of the radiator, arrange all sorts of objects around it and pretend that it was the driver's cab of a lorry. One of us would take the wheel and imitate the roar of the motor. That game was developed over the years as our knowledge of these matters increased. Later we fitted a steering wheel, made a dashboard of cardboard and a gear lever, while a hole punch served as an accelerator. We drove the lorry by turns until our mouths and throats were sore.

In my early memories my grandmother was always at my side. Her love for me was boundless but because of her character she could at times be very demanding. As the object of her overwhelming affection and concern I was constantly suspected of being ill, pining away, or perhaps lacking in appetite. My mother shared all these anxieties with her. Perhaps I did look ill; maybe my complexion was a little unhealthy. They thought that I was not sufficiently active and boisterous and were worried because it was not until I was almost three that I began to talk.

My grandmother watched over me to an almost embarrassing degree. She always came with me to the park and supervised my games; often interfering to help me beat the others. This was perhaps understandable but I disliked it and felt it unfair. As long as I can remember, my grandmother's interference and concern aroused a deep desire in me for independence which her persistence only aggravated.

My grandmother was a woman of strong passions. Her feelings were never temperate and her character was frequently unbearable. She remembered many of the proverbs and sayings popular in her village and used them regularly. Of herself she said that `she often burnt the house to get rid of the mouse' and I believe that she was absolutely right. Those whom she met through her life could never be accepted half-heartedly. They were either black or white; usually from the first meeting, and forever.

Perhaps because of this attitude it seemed to me that my grandmother was convinced from the very first moment I can remember that I was endowed with outstanding qualities. In her eyes I was handsome because I resembled her husband, Grandfather Slavcho and because of that I was also kind-hearted and noble in spirit despite being somewhat naive. It was the same characteristic traits that prevented her from liking my father and in our somewhat polarised domestic relationships my grandmother drew me very close to her in a way which undoubtedly established an emotional distance between me and my father.

My grandmother's impulsive reactions went beyond this. She had reached the conclusion that my brother resembled our father and showed some of his negative qualities. In her view the worst of these would be a tendency to profiteering and gluttony; the qualities she always associated with those she disliked. If I am to be fair I must admit that my grandmother was not entirely free of those same characteristics; nevertheless since birth my brother was measured by a different yardstick. While I was a poor eater my brother's excellent appetite supported Grandmother's suspicion that she was right in her judgement.

My father must never have been at ease in those years. His character was totally incompatible with my grandmother's. He was intelligent, good-mannered and clever; had a fine sense of humour and irony and a talent for mathematics and theoretical mechanics. He was a good mixer, weighed people up quickly and won his way into their heart. But behind his refined manner lay a nervous, hot-tempered and troubled man. His years in the army had developed a taste for ostentatious social life, for entertaining people and for visiting restaurants. That in itself was why he appreciated fine wines, spirits and haute cuisine and this was all the ammunition Grandmother needed to sustain her opposition to him.

I remember my father as an energetic and restless man who rose early. He was a keen philatelist. Every time that I approached to look at the stamp albums in which he arranged his collection I sensed that he was worried that I might sneeze or cough and damage them. I loved to examine the tiny pictures on the stamps and these always excited my imagination. Whenever my father was in a good mood he would talk to himself while arranging his stamps. This was the first occasion when I heard of Alsace and Lorraine. At the time they sounded to me like strange far-off places where life was different. I was not to know that forty years later, Lorraine would become my home.

My somewhat nervous and irritable father was carefully controlled in the family circle by my mother. She bridged the character, culture and personality differences between my father and grandmother and her patience and tact were exceptional. My mother was calm and well-balanced and did everything in her life with characteristic elegance and charm. She had an innate ability to transform all that she touched into something more beautiful, clean and orderly. She had refined, exquisite taste and was always smartly dressed. Wherever she moved she created harmony and beauty around her. Even the humble things of life such as arranging a bunch of flowers, laying the table, cooking or sewing were done in a special way. The most remarkable thing of all was that this behaviour was always natural, simple and spontaneous; seemingly without conscious effort.

I am not exaggerating when I say that my grandmother loved me more than any other person in her life. My mother loved me just as much, too. She unquestionably loved her other children but between the two of us there was a very special bond. Sometimes I found my grandmother impossibly irritating and overbearing and whereas she frequently got on my nerves, Mother and I lived in perfect harmony, loving each other with equal devotion. Perhaps it was that I loved her more than did her other children. We were deeply devoted to each other and it seemed that my mother had a sixth sense which enabled her to understand and feel all that happened to me, around me and within me despite the distance separating us.

When I was ill as a child nothing cheered me more than my mother's presence. At those times she would be so concerned with caring for me that she may have aroused my father's jealousy. He always said that I received too much attention and never missed the opportunity to make the point. My mother was accustomed to putting up with his temper and would calmly manage his regular outbursts for which there often appeared to be little justification. On the other hand he doted on her and could not bear being parted from her for even an instant. She was seldom angry with him but when she was, it was seriously so and took time to subside. Nevertheless they were a dedicated and happy couple.

Among all my childhood relatives and friends the most gentle and patient was my grandfather Slavcho. Despite being married to my volatile grandmother he himself was a quiet and calm man. He might perhaps be criticized for his undue fondness for cheap wine but he worked very hard indeed and I saw him only on Sundays. He rose early in the morning to take the train to Kazichene and came home late in the evening. To us small boys, Kazichene was very far away. Whenever we had an object or a person in our games who had to be dispensed with, they were sent to Kazichene. Grandfather would take us for a walk or a sleigh ride depending on the weather conditions. When we were tired he sat on a bench and perched us on his knee. I remember his palms bearing the marks of his craft; large, bony hands with rough skin tinted brown by the chemicals used in the leather industry. He would silently stroke my hair and I sensed his great love for me which I returned in full measure.

Family and Childhood

During my early childhood, life must have been very difficult for my family but nevertheless to me the world was full of love and perhaps that is why everything seemed beautiful and happy. The City Garden, a small park in front of the Czar's palace, was a hundred metres from our apartment. My mother or grandmother would take us there and my brother and I were fortunate indeed to spend so much time in one of Sofia's most beautiful places. It seemed that in the summer everything was green; there were big chestnut trees along the sandy paths and benches on each side. When we were still very young Mother or Grandmother would watch over us closely and we seemed to be allowed very few contacts with other children. However the games, the sunlight and the green foliage of the park remain in my memory as truly happy moments.

At the beginning of the 1950s, after the upheavals and the repression imposed to reinforce the newly-established Communist system, it seemed that a period of superficial stability would prevail. The acute shortages and rationing of earlier years disappeared. At the same time it was known that thousands were tortured or beaten to death in concentration camps such as those in Belene and Lovech, but we knew very little about these things and people were naturally reluctant to discuss them. There were taboos in my small boy's world; for example the Soviet Union had to be pronounced *USSR* as in the Latin alphabet and not as in the Bulgarian when it unfortunately sounded rude.

The dramatic change in my father's circumstances must have been a severe blow. After the initial period when he lived in fear of Communist repression he gradually adjusted to the new conditions like so many others. At the end of the 1940s, after graduating as a civil engineer, he briefly gained the approval of the Communist regime and was able to obtain employment. By that time, having used the pretext of *class struggle* to justify the destruction of the bourgeoisie the government was confronted with a shortage of educated and qualified people since so many of them were from this hated group. Certain army officers who had been dismissed were encouraged to return to service because their knowledge and education would enable them to train new recruits to the armed forces.

My father was now able to obtain a position with the Telegraph and Postal Institute; a semi-military body supported by the Post Office. He was happy once more to be in uniform although he would only keep his rank of captain for just a few more years. His feeling of being back in the service as an army officer was a short-lived illusion; he was in fact purely a teacher. Military training at the Institute came to an end after 1953 and my father stayed there teaching mathematics and theoretical mechanics until his eventual retirement.

My parents now had a better life as a result of father's new job. They were able to resume entertaining and dining out with old friends including my father's former colleagues from the Military School.

One of the family's closest friends was Vladi Udrev - my Uncle Vladi. He made a tremendous impression on me because of his charm, high education and intelligence; his brilliant sense of humour and boundless energy. Beyond this he owned a motorcycle, a prewar 125cc DKW. I was always happy to see his smiling face and to listen to his witty conversation. He had two charming daughters; Adriana, a year older than I, and Rosalina about a year younger. His wife was also extremely charming and intelligent and their daughters were brought up in a very free and open way.

Vladi Udrev owned a small company for the production of fire-fighting devices. It had been nationalised a couple of years earlier but he had been allowed to stay on as technical director which was common practice in those years of state appropriation of private companies. The Udrevs owned a comfortable and pleasant house in Poduene, a residential area in Sofia. I can still remember their spacious, immaculate kitchen with its beige and white tiles because it was there for the first time that I saw and handled Meccano, that system for the young engineer of metal pieces that could be assembled with nuts and bolts.

Uncle Vladi was a regular guest at home. My father began to work for him - earning a little extra by making drawings of the fire extinguishers, nozzles and hose reels manufactured by his firm. I could watch my father at work with pen and ink drawing at his board for hours if he would allow me. Our families often spent evenings together, although my brother and I would be sent to bed unless Adriana and Rosalina were invited too. Then we young folk would form a separate party. That always made me happy despite my childish prejudice against girls. I was about six years old at the time and liked Adriana a lot - she was rather free and even perhaps a little aggressive in her attitude to me. She seemed more mature than I and the difference in age was a sensitive issue at that time because I was ambitious to get the better of her. Rosalina was a charming little girl but she was of no real interest to me.

Our families spent the summer in the Vitosha mountains near Boyana. My father's institute organised a military training camp there and Uncle Vladi had a summer cottage nearby. These places remain in my memory as a paradise of lush meadows and green forests where we all lived together as one family. I can say, with nostalgia perhaps, that those were the happiest days of my childhood.

In the Vitosha meadows a game of pirates was organised for us four children. With the help of our parents, wooden knives were carved and a great rivalry in strength, agility and speed began. Adriana and Rosalina were real tomboys and combat was in their blood. Adriana was without question the best because she was the oldest, strongest and most mature. It was Adriana who would climb highest in the trees and throw stones further than any of us and we found it extremely difficult to beat her in any way. Each day she won another game and with that my childish heart.

I was very fond of my Uncle Vladi too. His disregard of the restrictions and precautions to which I was so accustomed, astonished me. Whenever Grandmother's common sense held me back, Vladi would say `let the boy see for himself whether it's right'. For example, I was told that eating maggoty cherries was unhealthy for me. Uncle Vladi then extracted a little worm from a cherry, calmly ate it and pronounced it excellent.

But it was really my Uncle Vladi's motorcycle that fascinated me most of all. I can vividly recall a summer day when he was adjusting the engine. The DKW was placed against the wall of the grassy yard and the black paint on its mudguards was warm to my touch. I inhaled and loved the aroma of petrol mixed with oil evaporating in the intense heat. From time to time my uncle Vlady would start the little two-stroke engine and the noise, vibrations and clouds of blue smoke from the exhaust pipe intoxicated me. My heart beat faster as he put me on the tank in front of him, placed my hands on the grips and kick-started the engine for me so that I could feel myself in charge.

Adriana intrigued me yet more and more and my ambition to dominate her absorbed all my waking thoughts. How was it that she could win all the games, just like a boy? For me this was paradoxical since I assumed that she considered that all women were like her. If women also gave birth to children, what was the purpose of men? At that time I had no understanding whatsoever of sex and I did not know how women became pregnant. In my

Family and Childhood

imagination I sought arguments to persuade Adriana of the importance of the male role in life. In my naive ignorance I was seriously mistaken, for Adriana knew very well the role of man, still unrevealed to me, because Uncle Vladi and his wife had intelligently initiated both daughters into the mysteries of sex and procreation.

It was much later that I realised how Adriana's understanding of nature differed so much from my own ideas. In the world of children playing pirates, where our rivalry surfaced, I was confronted by many strange new questions. Once while I was quietly urinating, Adriana came along and watched me in her characteristic open way. I did not regard this as a hostile act but was somewhat embarrassed. Nevertheless I vaguely suspected that my Uncle Vladi would not reproach her for her candour. I took my problem to Mother for advice and both she and Father laughed out loud. I heard them commenting out loud to each other that Adriana and Rosalina had been initiated into *everything* by their parents. What was that - *everything*? My parents would not tell me.

By the end of the summer Adriana had won my little boy's heart. I had eyes only for her when we were together. I can still remember her exact profile with small pointed chin and short straight fair hair silhouetted against the sun's rays seeping through the leaves. When we came home I thought only of her and dreamed constantly of meeting her again. Something had happened to me that was not of a child's world.

In the city park a mausoleum was built for the recently deceased Party Leader Georgi Dimitrov and at night mysterious greenish lights flickered behind its columns. The very idea that inside this building lay the mummified body of a man was depressing and somewhat frightening to us and we did not enjoy playing in that part of the park. From time to time I had nightmares in which the mausoleum featured prominently.

Suddenly my grandfather Slavcho fell ill and died of a severe infection in hospital within a fortnight. My grandmother cried heart-rendingly in a manner that I have never seen before or since.

Then something terrible happened to Uncle Vladi. At first my parents were so terrified that they were unable to tell me what it was or to hide their overwhelming fear. I could only catch snatches of what they said. It seemed that Vladi Udrev had been arrested, sentenced to death and summarily executed within ten days on charges of treason and spying - a common formula used to get rid of those considered hostile to the regime. I remember the tearful, tormented face of his widow sitting in our drawing room to tell us of her last meeting with him. He had informed her of the day when he would be executed and had asked her to be strong for the sake of the children. His wife and daughters were sent into exile to a village near the Danube. In later years he and his family would be rehabilitated. All of them remained forever in my memory and sometimes in my dreams, but I never saw them again.

I think that this was truly the end of my childhood.

Chapter Two
Those long school years

It was natural that my grandmother Stoena should accompany me on my first day at school. She waited outside until classes ended so that she could escort me home. If she had had the opportunity she would undoubtedly have peered through the windows to observe me at my desk in the classroom, but I do not remember seeing her.

From the very beginning the children in Comrade Ovcharova's class were pressed to compete for the very best results. We had come to this three-storey building - the Sixth Secondary Mixed School - that had been constructed at the turn of the century for the teaching of reading, writing, singing and drawing. The long mosaic-floored corridors polished smooth by the footsteps of generations of children were an ideal place to slide. The trill of a shrill electric bell was used to restore order among squabbling boys during the regular breaks.

Girls were expected to be paragons of good manners and diligence and were not expected to interfere in the friendships and activities of the boys. It was assumed that the two sexes were at war and if a boy mixed with the girls he became an object of derision. Physical superiority was important and the pecking order was quickly established. I resisted any attempt by my grandmother to protect me and was soon ranked among those capable of taking on anyone. My performance in lessons was adequate but in drawing I immediately became first in the class.

During my first year at school I met Boris Staykov. He arrived a few weeks after the rest of us since he had had an appendectomy. His mother introduced him to us as a distant cousin on my father's side of the family although this was unimportant since it was entirely up to us whether or not we hit it off. Boris was a sturdy tall boy with a relaxed nature and an intelligent mind. Bobby as we knew him lived with his mother and his grandparents. His parents were divorced and he seldom saw his father. His mother was an intelligent well-mannered and energetic lawyer. The family came from Macedonia and Bobby had something of that region's fighting spirit and never let down anyone spoiling for a fight regardless of the likely outcome. It was foreign to his nature to complain and he always made the most of any situation in which he found himself.

Bobby and I shared a desk and quickly became bosom pals regardless of the competitive spirit between us that endured for years. But there was also a feeling of mutual understanding and we discussed everything of interest. In the school atmosphere of that day this was extremely important to us.

At school the Soviet experience went far beyond the introduction of black uniforms and the hideous lilac ink which I hated. Songs in praise of Stalin followed lessons dedicated to extolling his greatness. Comrade Ovcharova taught us all about the basic features of the communist system - how to report on others and to speak ill of one's neighbour at the slightest opportunity. There was a lesson about a conscientious Soviet boy who denounced his parents to the authorities because they had hidden sacks of wheat. We never learned what actually happened to them but the moral of the story was that those prepared to betray their parents would be among the first to be welcomed into the Communist Youth Organisation, the Comsomol. I still remember vividly how Comrade Ovcharova declared in her most serious voice that there was a central secret file on each one of us in which everything that we said or did was faithfully recorded and which would be kept by the authorities for the rest of our lives.

It must therefore have been during my first year at school that the Roumen Antonov file was opened. Facing the class, I was asked whether I believed in God. Since I replied in the affirmative I must have committed the most heinous of crimes. I was immediately punished so that I could draw the necessary conclusions and my mother was summoned to see my teacher. Instead my father arrived in his captain's uniform which probably set Comrade Ovcharova's mind at ease. Army uniforms were now based on the Soviet model and Czarist swords had been abolished.

My school was in the city centre and all Party functionaries of importance lived nearby. A couple of children of such influential parents were present in my class and they were regarded very favourably in the school rankings. As our teacher was a model of obsequiousness her attitude to children depended very much on their social and political background. My father's uniform could not deceive her shrewd observation; my mother's religiosity, my father's background as a former Czarist officer and our relatives in the United States blighted my reputation and I was soon obliged to come to terms with that fact and to learn to live with it.

I cannot remember the exact moment when the teaching of my school and my own innermost thoughts parted company, never to meet again. Communist ideology was so all-pervasive at school that there was no room to consider whether to accept or reject it. Good and evil were defined on Stalin's principle that *anyone not with us must be against us*. At such an early age it was difficult to side with evil even if good was not always attractive. We were extremely young and a reprimand or praise would make a great impact on us. On matters concerned with mathematics and grammar our teacher had indisputable authority. However, I found myself rebelling unconsciously on every occasion when she expressed her displeasure with my lack of expression in the obligatory recital of poetry. I recall how one of my classmates with eyes closed and in a trance sang a song about Stalin at a school festival. Cold shivers went up and down my spine and I was delighted that I could not sing as he could. I was about nine when Stalin died and many of my classmates burst into tears - sincere tears, I am sure - when they heard the tragic voice of the newsreader echoing from the loudspeakers in the streets. My father could hardly suppress his jubilation and I wholeheartedly shared his feelings.

My friendship with Bobby helped us both to tolerate the most difficult lesson of our schooldays; that intended to teach us hypocrisy. We were expected to show our unbounded approval of all communist dogma and to express our reverence for Stalin and the other leaders. The degree of exultation expressed was carefully measured by our teacher and in the confined world of school it was judged to be the only standard of good and evil. In that unbalanced, traumatic atmosphere my friendship with Bobby gave comfort and support to us both. It was only with Bobby that I was able to express my true feelings and opinions. We were as millions of people under the yoke of Communism in that we could only reveal our true feelings to one or two of our closest friends. We soon discovered that we shared a fascination for the world of proscribed thought, books, objects and even individual words that blossomed forth from the point where Soviet communism ended.

Those long school years

Our first major discovery was books. I can still remember reading books with the grammar and spelling of the Czarist era. My favourites were the works of Jules Verne. By seeking refuge in the make-believe world of pirates and adventurers we were able to widen our horizons to foster ideas that were either ignored or forbidden by the school authorities. The subconscious fear of repression filling the atmosphere around us gave sincerity and romanticism to our preferences. Among the characters we found fascinating there was not a single one with a Russian name and certainly none of those appearing in the approved list of books for required reading.

When we played chess which was often, Bobby usually won. We also played with tin soldiers that acted as the people of our imaginary world. Jules Verne's books kindled our imagination and we had long discussions about science and technology as they appeared to our young boys' minds. Bobby's grandfather was a retired schoolmaster who acted as a source of encyclopaedic reference on any subject which aroused our curiosity. We often discussed history and the events of the Second World War. Our common interests and discussions that began during the first school year gradually broadened in the years to come.

I think that I fell in love for the first time in those early years at school.

The girl who was the subject of my admiration increasingly attracted my attention and gradually took a firm place in my heart and mind. She was a classmate and the daughter of an Establishment communist poet. Naturally she was one of the very best students and I was unable to have more than a few contacts with her and it was only the beauty that I imagined her to have that fascinated me. Natural beauty was a quality that I greatly appreciated; it would always excite me just as its presence would continue to make me feel ill at ease throughout my life. This first infatuation resulted in a four line poem written at the age of eleven. Sadly the girl of my dreams failed to show any great interest in me.

On 20 January 1952, one day before my eighth birthday, my sister Violet was born. The family still shared a flat with the Ikonomovs. Mr Ikonomov was a quiet man but his wife Vasilka was aggressive in nature and cunning in her behaviour; which my grandmother could not tolerate. To be obliged to live with another family was a constant source of friction and each group felt deprived by the other of its privacy and then took advantage of the situation. Beneath a thin, superficial layer of politeness lay a tension that often erupted in brawls between Vasilka and my grandmother. The Ikonomov's daughter was bullied by her mother and my brother and I bore her little respect. Her brother we found to be a quiet, easy-going lad.

We felt that there was no hope that our family living conditions might ever improve. Nevertheless my parents lived happily together and loved and doted on us children. My father had a patriarchal disposition and loved to have us all around him at dinner in the shared drawing room. He enjoyed the evenings and could disregard my grandmother's customary iciness and the continual coming and goings of the Ikonomovs while we were having dinner.

When seated at the head of the table Father was entirely in his element. He enjoyed leading the conversation and giving instructions on how to serve the dishes while at the same time making sarcastic comments about the Ikonomovs passing through the room or on Grandmother's response to them. We frequently travelled out of town for a picnic and my mother would make delicious sandwiches to take with us. In the summer my grandmother would usually take us to the seaside and our holidays customarily ended with a visit to her native village of Dolni Lozen.

My brother and I shared a few toys. Gradually all pre-war toys disappeared and the meagre range of toys on sale in the shops did little to arouse our interest. The best we managed was a toy truck for me and a single-seater racing car for my brother, both made of metal and with a clockwork mechanism wound up by a protruding key. They came from the Czechoslovakian shop in Sofia and for a long time these two vehicles and the tin soldiers were our favourite toys. Later I painted the now chipped lorry bright red. I remember my sister Violet as a toddler eager to join us in playing with the lorry and the lined up soldiers but we would not allow this; she was too young and after all she was just a girl.

Above us on the third floor lived the Georgiev family. Sadly their daughter had died after giving birth to a son Georgi. His father remarried and Georgi was brought up by a stepmother who was as evil as the classic fairy-tale version. Georgi and his parents lived in Poduene and he often came to visit the grandparents, seeking comfort away from the cheerless home with a father who did not care for him. I could not help overhearing my parents saying that his stepmother's dislike of him sometimes turned into simple cruelty.

We befriended Gosho as we called him at the time. Whenever he visited his grandparents he made a point of coming downstairs to see us. The three of us together formed the first group to which parental access was firmly denied. By defying adult taboos my brother and I were soon acquainted with the secrets of life and adopted the obscene words Gosho had learned in the streets of Poduene. The secret use of indecent expressions and foul language soon became for us a competitive activity and we quickly mastered the art of cursing. Gosho indulged in wild fantasies of sexual relations in which reality and fiction blended seamlessly. We often laughed at him for his crazy stories.

Gosho would frequently run away from his stepmother's cruelty to seek comfort with his grandparents. I was about ten when a shocking incident took place. His stepmother hit him with a hot poker and his grandparents were so upset by this that they insisted that he should come and live with them. This brought us closer together and he became part of my family group. The three of us spent every day together with Gosho initiating all kinds of games using marbles and cards or what we called *flower planting;* a game played by arranging coloured glass marbles and pieces of mosaic in various patterns. As he put so many of his infectious feelings and passions into these games Gosho soon became the most essential part of them; without him taking part they seemed tedious. Once whilst arguing he called himself Shego instead of Gosho and this new name stuck to him for the rest of his life.

We gradually formed a large group as some of the neighbourhood children joined us in our games in the City Garden. Some were my classmates. Under the influence of the movie of *The Three Musketeers* we fashioned rapiers from iron rods and tin boxes and began to duel. Our playground was situated before the Exhibition Hall which replaced the former Sofia Casino and the Czarist City Hall where the Comsomol Organisation was now based. Between these two buildings was a small patch of grass which we conquered and regarded as our play area for many years.

This was the place where three aged photographers still practised their art. They took pictures using what appeared to be a wooden box on a tripod with an old Agfa camera inside it. Two tiny drawers contained boxes of chemical and after a couple of minutes of rapid manipulation the photographer would thrust his hand into a long black fabric sleeve and extract a dripping picture of dubious quality. These three old photographers became our devoted friends and patrons. The eldest among them was a short thin man called

Those long school years

Uncheto who resembled Lenin with his cap and shabby jacket with tie permanently in place. He outlived his colleagues and continued to take pictures late into the 1960s when some of the boys were already married. Years later whenever we observed him still appearing healthy and energetic, he told us that the secret lay in eating grilled liver and kidneys.

At our secondary school Shego and I were in the same class. As usual it was the personality of our teachers that could make us enjoy or hate individual classes. We found mathematics hard to learn and many disliked it. On the contrary, history and geography we found easy and stuffed with *class definitions* intended to enlighten us. Biology was the same with all the absurdities dreamed up by the Soviet biologists Michurin and Lisenko who had rejected the theories of genetics. It seemed to us that the only function of physics was to bolster the communist dogma that the *motion of matter* was the driving force of everything in our world. The Russian language was taught intensively and I found music classes an absolute nightmare. I always found difficulty in literature classes since we were required to write essays based on dogma and as a relief from this boring activity to recite the output of communist poets. Short hair was mandatory and all Western fashions in music and behaviour were outlawed, with older students even being sent to labour camp as punishment for innocently wearing excessively tight trousers.

A Russian book entitled *Povest ob Avtomobyle* (The Story of the Car) had a great influence. It was filled with monochrome drawings of the few cars manufactured in the Soviet Union together with sectioned drawings of engines, transmissions, differentials and other mechanical parts. I soon grasped the principles described rather modestly in this book and in my imagination the Otto 4-cycle engine began to run as it would continue to do throughout my life. This book failed to convince me that the Russians held the lead as inventors of engines or as leaders of car manufacture with Stalin at the head (as seemed to be the intention of the introduction). Nevertheless it gave me an understanding of the spiritual and cultural iron curtain behind which I found myself enclosed even in the case of these wonderful vehicles that had captured my imagination.

The universe of Western cars beyond the Soviet models with which I was now familiar glittered in vague shapes and colours in my imagination stimulated by the occasional advertisements and photographs sent to me from America by my Aunt Tanya. The Soviet Pobedas gradually came to dominate the streets of Sofia and formed humdrum processions of identical shapes in their dull beige paintwork, just occasionally but ever infrequently disrupted by the few remaining prewar cars that remained in circulation.

I began to collect photographs and drawings of cars and motorcycles. Books and magazines with such illustrations of complete cars or their components became my cherished possessions and I was prepared to swap any other treasures for these. I remember the tiny coloured pictures of cars contained in chocolate wrappings during the 1950s and I managed to obtain a dozen of these in exchange for a pair of tin soldiers and the pocket money intended for my daily snack.

In the autumn of 1956 a short newspaper article made a profound impression on me. Something was happening in Budapest that was described as a riot by criminals. Very soon the Hungarian Revolution began to grasp my attention and to absorb my emotions. Like my father, many people observed these events in minute detail. In the evening we gathered around our prewar wireless set and listened to the reports of Radio Free Europe and the Voice of America despite the heavy jamming by local special equipment. At times we were able to tune to these stations and listen to them with reasonable clarity. At other times we had to guess the meaning of words fading away in the drone of the jammers. Tension increased in Sofia too. For the first time in my life I witnessed the violence of the spoken word as a policeman in plain clothes reached for the gun hidden under his jacket and yelled `Come on, just try and I'll show you, you filthy scum.' He was probably addressing an anonymous passer-by in the crowd after overhearing a gratuitous insult.

Millions of Hungarians were caught up in the terror in their country. After the crushing of the Hungarian Revolution I continued to listen daily to the news bulletins, hanging on every word. My father no longer wished to join me but would occasionally ask about the situation.

At the end of 1959 I heard during one of the forbidden broadcasts a reference to the demonstration of a new type of internal combustion engine in New York. This was the creation of Felix Wankel and was lighter and smaller than conventional engines thanks to its rotating piston mechanism. I can remember vividly that precise moment as I sat pressing my ear against the dusty grille of the wireless speaker with the glowing valves inside the wooden case emitting their characteristic smell. This news made a great impression on me and I was immediately curious to know precisely how Wankel's engine worked. My imagination had been challenged to work out how the rotating piston functioned - this was quite beyond my experience. Months later a diagram and brief description of the Wankel engine were published in a magazine and as I tried to understand its principles I felt myself beginning a long journey of discovery. From that point on I became dominated by the desire to invent an even more advanced internal combustion engine. It became a long and complicated story.

In the small corner of the City Garden where I played with other boys from the neighbourhood the world was quite different. We shouted obscene words at each other; won and lost countless games of marbles and Shego pursued his lonely interest in the collection of cigarette boxes. Wankel and his engine were no longer an interesting topic of discussion. The aged photographers ogled every attractive girl passing by and their comments began to open up a new world to us. We still felt superior about girls but our interest in the opposite sex was growing.

One summer a pretty girl with red hair and green eyes came to the park with a little boy. Mariana was my age - fourteen - and had small pointed breasts within her tight blouse. As a newcomer she did not seem embarrassed by us and I found myself accepting her as an equal. My friends showed her respect and when she was near us filthy language was never used. Mariana observed me with her imperturbable smile and one day I approached her and told her I was prepared to do something with her. She did not seem to be shocked and asked me to tell her exactly what I meant. When I told her that I wished to make love to her she blushed but did not seem angry and looked away with a quiet laugh. We continued to flirt with the same frankness for some time until Mariana accused me of never going beyond mere words. She seemed willing but we had nowhere to go. It's difficult for me to say whether I felt true love but Mariana was indeed the first girl who aroused strong and distinct sexual desire in me. Perhaps our conversation was just outrageously rejecting the aspects of communist ideology that considered sex to be mere bourgeois decadence. But this small corner in the City Garden was part of a free country which we had declared a long time ago.

Bobby and I continued our youthful discussions through the spiritual and emotional stages of puberty. We would often take long walks in the better parts of the city lost in conversation about the world and the future, about politics, technology and our fellow human beings. It was during that period that Kruschev began the process of criticizing Stalin and of taking steps to liberalise the Soviet system into a less repressive regime. The period of détente stimulated our yearning to embrace the civilization denounced as decadent during our childhood. In our youthful enthusiasm we dreamed of an open road before us and at the threshold of this unknown future we felt beautiful moments when we dreamed of travel and discovery in the huge unexplored world around us. Such feelings dominated the summer holidays we spent with our parents in Varna, the Black Sea seaside resort which had for many years been re-named *Stalin* but had now reverted to its original Czarist name. Bobby's mother had now re-married and he had a little sister.

Our new hobby was photography. I bought a Soviet Russian camera; a 6x6cm Bakelite box of poor quality. I taught myself to make contact prints directly on to photographic paper that I developed and fixed myself. The result was frankly uninspiring and we later bought a very cheap East German camera with an even worse lens than its Russian predecessor. Our attempts to print the photographs using a primitive enlarger were even less successful and our hobby came to an end with only a few snapshots of poor quality remaining. We did not allow this to ruin the many happy hours that we spent in search of interesting subjects to photograph. Under my leadership Bobby combed the quieter streets of the capital in pursuit of pre-war motor cars as subject matter.

Another of our hobbies, cycling, was also disastrous. A bicycle formed part of my dream of transport on wheels and eventually my Grandmother suppressed her dread of an accident and gave in to my persistent requests for help. She eventually agreed to buy me a Yugoslavian bicycle and Bobby's mother bought him exactly the same model. Together we had great fun riding round the streets of Sofia and travelling out into the suburbs. But sadly these rather primitive bicycles often broke down until finally we found it impossible to repair them.

I befriended Branimir Vidinski, a classmate. He was a good-looking and sensitive boy of high intelligence, with good manners. There was a finesse and vitality in his character which was quite different from the phlegmatic Bobbie. I too felt myself sometimes rather awkward and slow in Branimir's company but we were nevertheless the best of friends. It was Branimir who introduced me to amateur radio. We joined a club and began to make simple radio receivers with a crystal to pick up the signal and a manually wound coil. The whole assembly was mounted on a piece of plywood. One evening my efforts were rewarded when I succeeded in picking up some Russian folk music somewhat overshadowed by an irritating and piercing background noise. My second radio receiver was fitted with a radio valve but this did nothing to improve the quality of the reception. I finally abandoned my experiments with radio waves and concentrated on motor cars. Years later it was my turn to introduce Branimir to my own favourite hobby, car engines.

One of my favourite books at the time was *The Adventures Of The Good Soldier Svejk During World War I* by the Czech writer Jaroslav Hasek. I read and re-read this book many times and can recall certain passages to this very day. Its impact remains a mystery to me but without question it has made me laugh more than anything else in the world. To many of us living behind the Iron Curtain it offered a means of tolerating the system - by mocking its cruelty and absurdities. Hasek's magic had a similar impact on Bobby and most of my friends and we developed a secret code of words and phrases based on the book. Ten years later when the Czech Spring was brutally crushed by Soviet tanks the entire book was read on the radio in Czechoslovakia. Svejk was our bible and helped us to laugh off violence against the human mind. I owe it a great deal.

At the end of the Fifties the total isolation of the Communist bloc began to relax and certain writers were translated into Bulgarian. Books by Remarque, Steinbeck and Hemingway were difficult to find and I enthusiastically read anything I could track down. I read all the books that the Western literature section of the Sofia city library could offer and soon it became difficult to find a book that I did not already know well. Bobby and I exchanged all the books that we could find and our ideas of the real world outside our borders were formed through the eyes of their characters, mostly young immigrants in Paris who spent their time drinking Calvados and quietly mocking their misfortunes in love and the appalling chaos of life in general. We became totally absorbed in the atmosphere of these books and came to imitate our favourite characters. Ironically this experience became part of my own life thirty years later.

As fifteen year-old students at the high school we now wore depressing dark blue uniforms and caps. The girls wore black pinafores and berets. We had now suddenly grown up into adolescents, our voices had broken and our idealism was not yet fully formed. The girls had become significantly prettier and most of them were very feminine under the shining sateen of their black dresses. The change caused us to nervously seek our new personalities. I was no less confused than the others but probably more ambitious in my competition with the other boys. My friend Bobby was in another class but Branimir and Shego were still with me.

Shego had had a difficult childhood and his youth was even more so. He was rather late in entering puberty and found that depressing. His grandparents had little money to spare for him and he felt himself the most poorly dressed boy of the class. Nevertheless he had a bright mind and vivid imagination but his depression caused him to become a shabby young man with little self-confidence. In order to compensate for his imagined appearance he became rather eccentric in manner and outrageously obscene in speech. Grubby and slovenly, Shego applied his powers of imagination to devise disgustingly filthy stories. Sometimes they would help him to attract the attention and approval of his classmates but more often than not they shocked those foolish enough to read them. I greatly enjoyed myself reading some of his pornography but I was mainly amused by his inexhaustible application and vigorous creativity. He was always on the point of failing his examinations since he devoted most of his time to filling notebooks with coloured drawings and descriptions of fantastic animals whose main activity was the discharge of excrement and revolting gases from the most improbable bodily outlets. These deformed creatures peopled his own country on the imaginary planet of *Cyrasculia* whose territory we had divided among ourselves long ago.

In his thick notebooks Shego kept comments on the activities in his country, consisting mainly of complicated games of dice. I had long ago abandoned my country on the planet Cyrasculia but for many years Shego, Bobby, my brother and friends would often assemble to organise Olympic Games that were great fun with numerous imaginary competitors bearing outrageously indecent names. Years later whenever I had a difficult time I would recall some of these names which never failed to make me laugh again.

Despite his shabbiness, Shego had a certain charm of manner which was nevertheless difficult for outsiders to appreciate. His determination to shock drove him to behave in the strangest way. At a later stage he began to write sentimental love poems that were nothing but lachrymose nonsense. They failed to secure the attention of girls but Shego nevertheless continued to enjoy writing them, producing his unpretentious text in huge volume.

My sister Violet was everybody's darling in those years. She was bright and kind-hearted and we got along very well together. She was without question my father's favourite and he showed much more affection to her than to me or my brother. That made my brother jealous and he complained that he was denied love and attention. But these were passing moods because he was by nature somewhat unstable, which also influenced his way

Those long school years

of making decisions. He would deliberate at length before undertaking anything and his indecisiveness grew stronger and stronger. For example he was the sort of person who could spend half an hour wondering whether he should go out with or without a hat. Having finally decided to emerge covered he would return five minutes later and remove his hat. Despite all this he had a sense of humour and was good at singing and playing the mouth organ. Later he decided to become a professional singer and passed hours on end locked in the bathroom imitating Harry Belafonte. He was an outstanding success singing indecent popular songs with Shego and other friends.

Although she had by now brought four children into the world and was approaching her fortieth birthday, my mother was still beautiful and passers-by would turn to look back at her in admiration. At the end of the 1950s she worked as a fashion model for the newly published women's magazines and clothes shows. Her impressive good looks were preserved into her old age and she was able to work as a model until she was sixty, with completely white hair. She received letters from many admirers and some of my classmates envied me my beautiful mother. My father would never allow her to travel alone to the numerous fashion shows out in the country, although Mother was faithful to him all her life without any apparent difficulty. She had given him her love forever; her life was settled and no other man or event would even temporarily disturb her. She read romantic novels but the passionate stories they contained never made her discontented. The songs of Edith Piaf which were permitted on Bulgarian State Radio aroused her emotions and she enjoyed listening to them. Whenever a Piaf song was played she put her work to one side and listened entranced to the very end of it. Yves Montand, the first singer from the West to visit Sofia after his successful Soviet tour won over my mother and me and we became his faithful fans for life.

My grandmother lived in a self-contained world of her own. Her tiny pension was never used for daily living expenses since she saved it to buy presents for me. She lived a life of sobriety and only succumbed to her hearty appetite if the food was provided by others. She liked wine and home-made brandy. Her manners were hardly polite and she never accepted advice from others. She was an extremely sturdy woman and her physical strength was not to be underestimated even at the age of sixty. One evening a drunkard tried to attack her in the entrance hall of our apartment. He must have regretted his action immediately as Grandmother felled him with a single blow and calmly walked past him up the stairs. Whenever involved in an argument in a shop she made sure that the outcome was in her favour. She loved flowers and her room was filled with numerous pot plants on which she lavished especial care. In her love for me the most irritating feature was her wish to watch over me in all aspects of my life which often amounted to outright spying. She was very sensitive to everything I said or did and if I was angry with her she would cry like an offended little girl. She would hide a piece of fruit, a cake or a sweet from my brother so that she could give it to me and would follow me about with a snack trying to persuade me to eat it.

The years that I spent at school seemed never-ending. The first day of the summer holidays was the most enjoyable moment for me. Summer was sunny and wonderful; life was devoid of uniforms, school rallies and parades. The tedious pattern of homework, arriving late at school and having my hair cut off gave way to more pleasant activities. During the summer we children gathered in our corner of the City Garden that was named Congo after the latest war in Africa during the 1950s. A couple of girls came along to join us and Shego fell hopelessly in love with one of them to whom he dedicated a collection of poems. Remarque's novels played an essential part in forming my emotional life and my true feelings were kept safe for an ideal, unusual blue-eyed utterly charming girl whom I never actually met. I thought that the girls who came to the park were foolish but some nevertheless attracted me sexually. Although our joint tenants' daughter let me fondle her in the narrow hall I was never truly in love with her. I dated some of the girls and took them for long walks in the city park where we would sit on a bench and kiss and cuddle but none of them won my heart. It was nice to know that girls liked me but my dream of a future idealised love intrigued me far more than an association with the real girls around me.

In my heart and mind there was room for another ideal love.

On the ground floor of the Central Department Store in the centre of Sofia there was a display of motor cars. These products of the Socialist world included the Moskvitch from the Soviet Union, the Skoda from Czechoslovakia, the Wartburg from East Germany and the French Renault 4CV. There were indeed few buyers since Socialist equality had made everyone poor and the price of 20,000 levs seemed decadently outrageous in a capitalist way. I often went to look over the cars and the adjoining motorcycles of Czech, East German and Soviet origin. To own one of them seemed to me a more realistic dream and I spent hours imagining how I might one day be able to afford a motorcycle probably after winning on the recently established national lottery. I dreamed of taking the shiny black MZ 125cc that was the postwar version of Uncle Vladi's motorcycle. The solid AWO machine modelled after BMW and equipped with a four-stroke engine was so overwhelmingly beautiful and costly that it seemed foolish to even dream of possessing it. On my way to the department store I always walked past the City Centre Hotel and sometimes I was lucky enough to glimpse a few of the Western cars that happened to be passing through Sofia.

At the age of fifteen I joined a motorcycling club which provided me with the opportunity to apply for a driving test. It was the first time that I had driven a vehicle; now actually feeling the engine under my control as I had dreamed all those years. Immediately after my sixteenth birthday I passed the test and got my driving licence. All I had to do now was to win the lottery and my dream would come true with the result that on the only time I won on the lottery I had bought three new tickets. Now my mania to own a motorcycle made my grandmother and mother extremely nervous as they were certain that one day I would have a serious accident. On one occasion I entered a motorcycle show with a Wall of Death and Loop the Loop. When I arrived home I found both Mother and Grandmother with red swollen eyes; a representative of the organisers had called on them with papers for their written permission to let me ride.

My favourite car at this time was the prewar Fiat 500 *Topolino* (little mouse). I was fascinated by its beautiful lines and small overall dimensions that made it seem slightly easier to possess. Whatever were its charms, every evening it was of the *Topolino* that I dreamed before falling asleep. In my dream I painted it black or red but always with a tint of light cream on the sides and the wheel rims and I equipped it with leather seats, a special dashboard and a radio. The more practical details of my intended purchase were left for the future.

When I finally did acquire a *Topolino* it was rather different from my imagining. In the real world of education, professional training classes were introduced and we were lucky to have among them lessons in motor car mechanics. The young inexperienced teacher soon had to accept my total competence in matters automotive. The school owned a

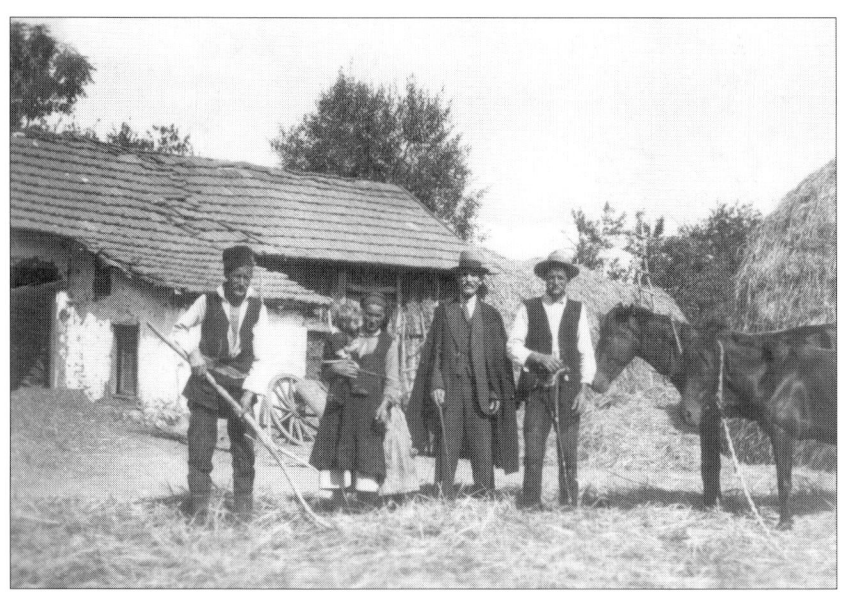

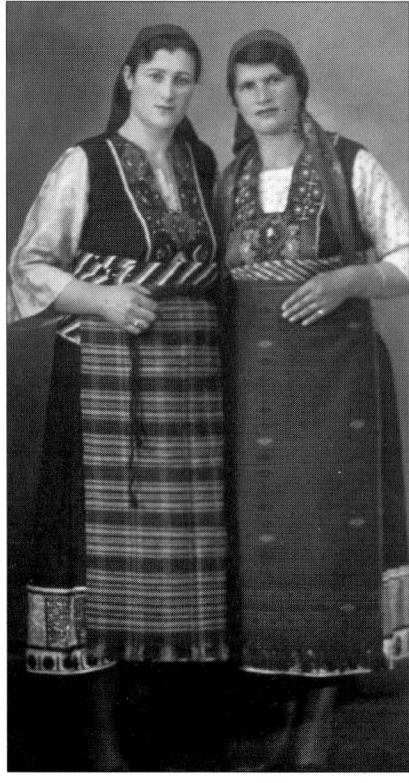

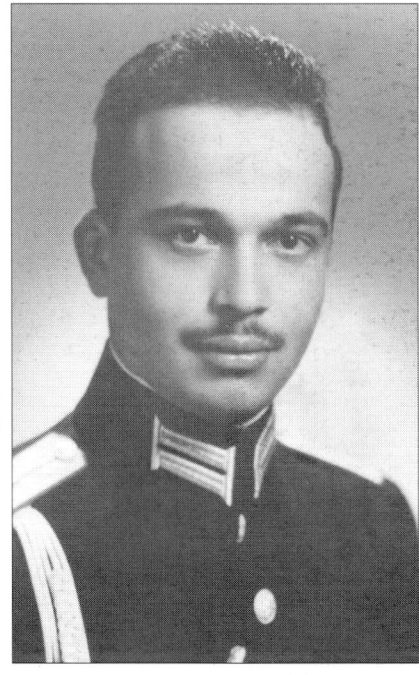

Grandmother's house in the village of Dolni Lozen, 1933 (top)

Grandmother Stoena (Left) and her sister in traditional Shopp costume (left)

My father Anton in the late Thirties (above)

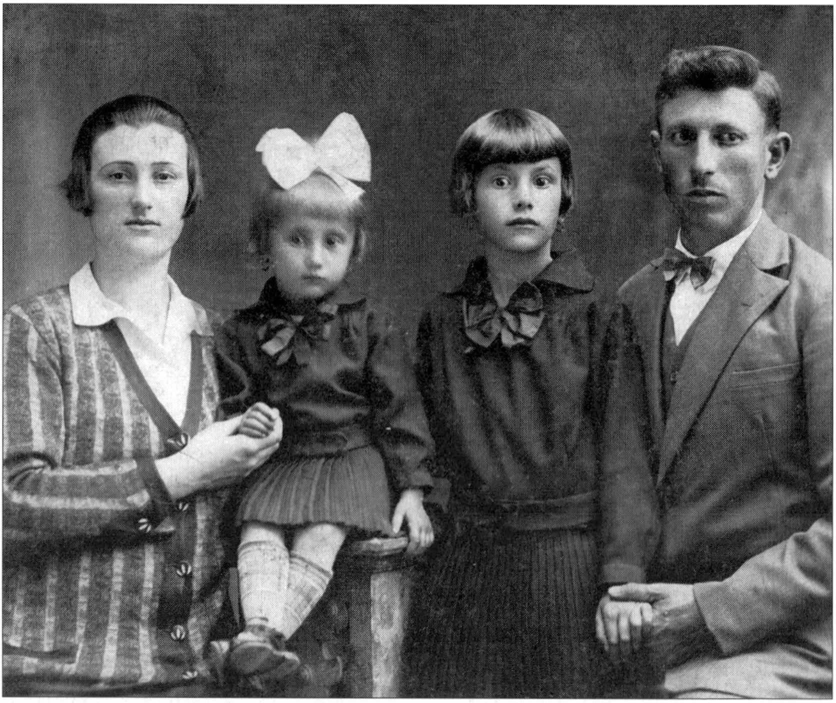

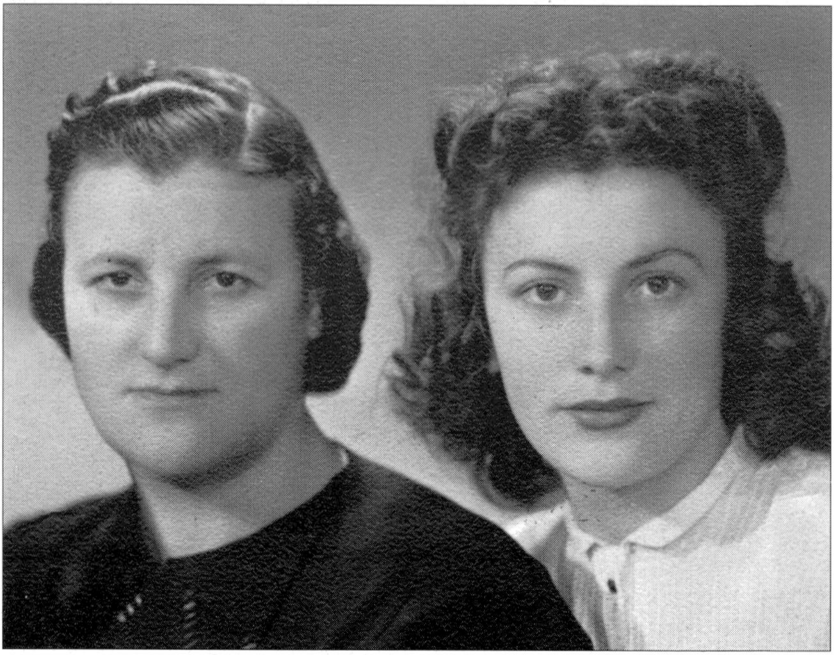

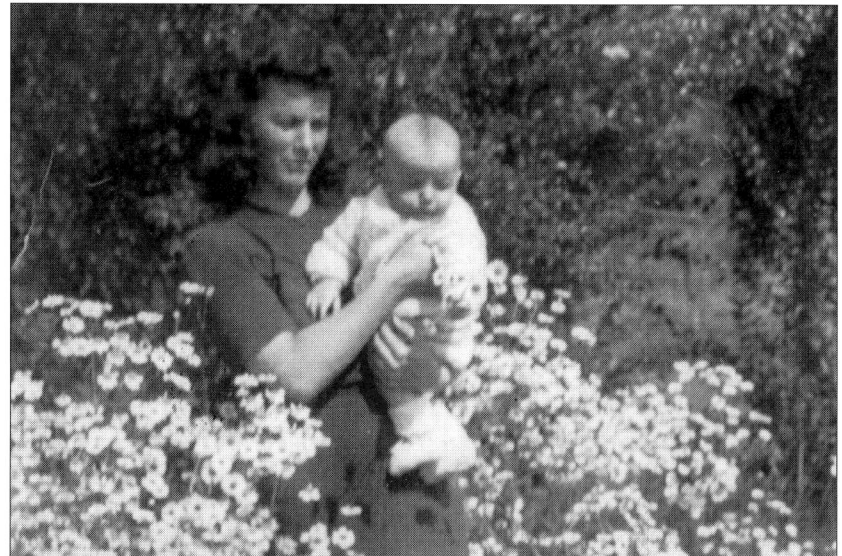

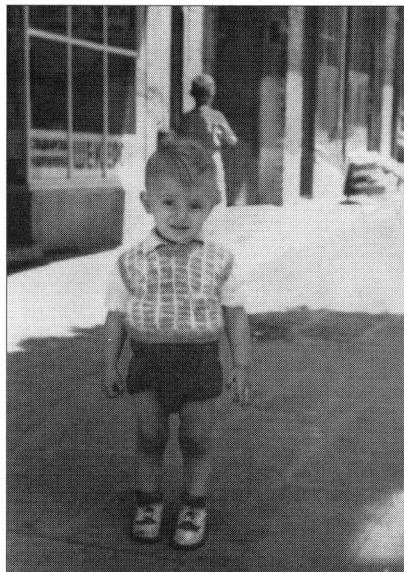

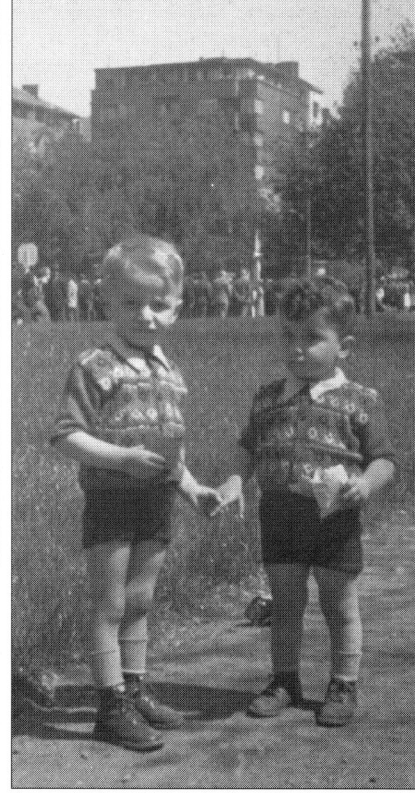

Grandmother's family in the late Twenties. (opposite left to right): Grandmother Stoena, her daughters Tanya and Evgenya and Grandfather Svetoslav

Grandmother and Mother at the end of the Thirties (opposite below)

Mother and I in spring 1944. During the Allied bombing of Sofia we were evacuated to the nearby village of Malo Bouchino (top)

The little street urchin of 1946 (above)

My brother Evgeni and I in the late Forties. One of the many parades held at that time can be seen in the background (right)

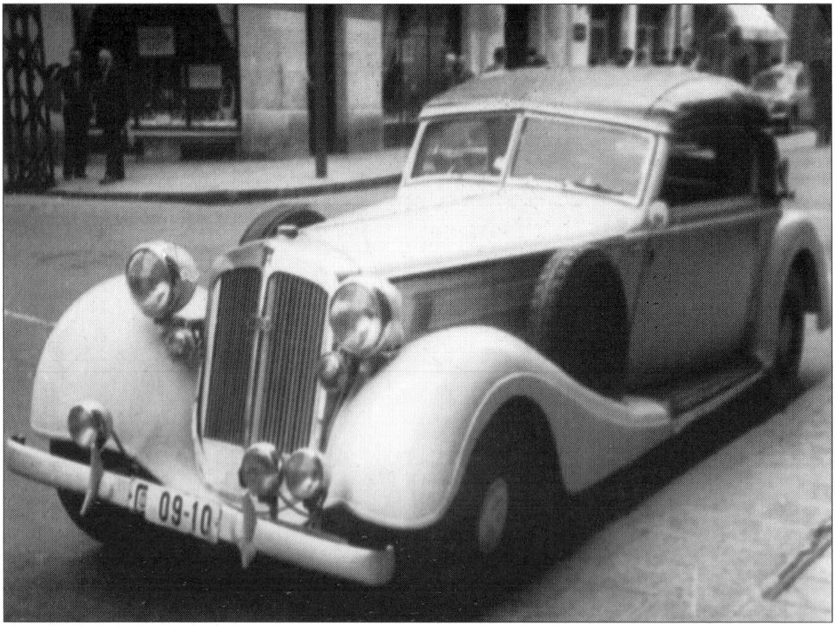

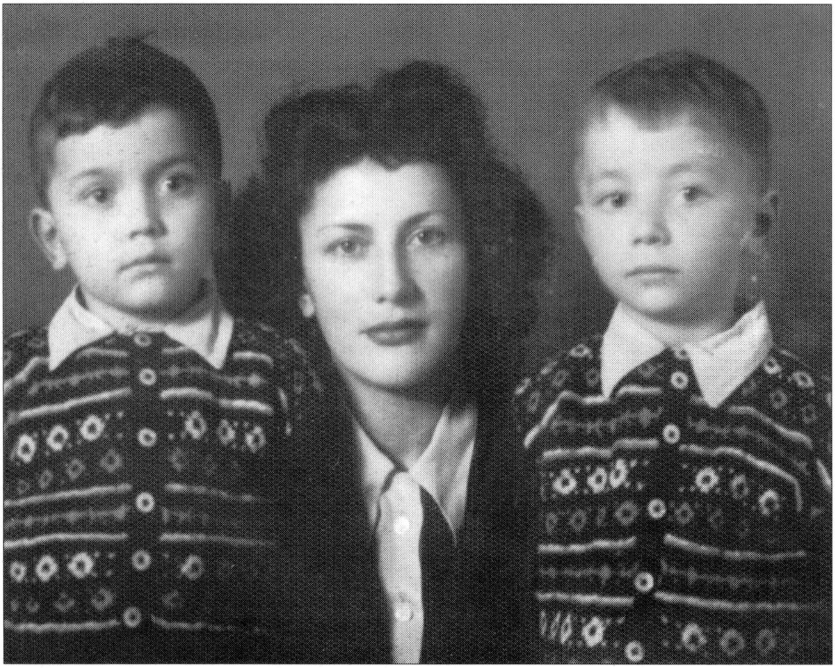

One of the cars that impressed me as a child, a Horch 853 often parked near our apartment (above)
Mother with my brother Evgeni (left) and me in 1950 (right)

Those long school years

Topolino for training purposes. It was in bad shape because its former owner had used it as a van and had installed a crude wooden platform behind the driver's seat. The car was painted in dull grey applied with a brush and the seats and interior were very grimy. But it was my first car and behind its small steering wheel I drove the first few hesitating metres of my life. Despite my great love for this car it could not be saved and was soon discarded on the large playing field behind the school above the atomic shelter. Other schoolchildren took it apart and destroyed it and I had to face the fact that it was now beyond repair. I constantly fiddled under the bonnet and sometimes spent hours behind the steering wheel dreaming of how one day I would have more good luck and the opportunity and wherewithal to restore it.

Reality and my ideas of motor cars fed by thoughts of the engine of Felix Wankel were worlds apart. I often considered the construction of a simpler engine than this. I do not remember at what age I made my first engine drawing but by sixteen I had already made many elaborate designs. My engine was hardly original and I seriously doubt if it had any advantage over the competition, but I loved drawing it. I came across the Russian translation of a collection of articles by German engineers with an important role at that historical period. The two volumes of *A Reference Book of Motor Cars* gave me a wide knowledge of the subject and became my faithful companion for many years. I ripped out and took one of its chapters with me when I emigrated to Paris thirty years later. In search of a new engine I incidentally invented new brakes, a chassis and transmission. In my science classes I even busied myself inventing a non-existent electric motor.

Descending the stairs on my way to school I frequently wondered what I would do in the future. I always saw myself working with cars but felt intuitively that there was something else of importance for me to do in the field of science. What was that unknown thing without pistons and of which I had not the faintest understanding at this time? I once said to Shego as we went downstairs that one day I would discover some vital medical innovation. At the time of course he refused to believe me but twenty years later I invited him to test my medical theories.

Once at street level I walked on my way to school. Eleven years of strolling along the same pavement seemed a very long time to me and I was eager to reach the end of the road where I imagined real life to begin. I sought feverishly the idols of my dreams but they often turned out to be snobbish frauds who flattered me with their oily manners. Emotions awakened by strange new experiences made the world around me an unreal place of frustrating contacts. I was strongly attracted to a girl in my class but her narrow and petty personality became an irritation. I arrogantly ignored the attention of other girls and was then confused by the avid declarations of love made to me by a school beauty who dazzled me with her very presence.

Many changes took place in me during my last school year when I was seventeen. All the higher classes of the Sixth School were moved into another school. There was a different atmosphere and new teachers and classmates changed my world profoundly. Suffering from the distortion of endless copyings and re-recordings, Elvis Presley's rock and roll sounded hollow as it emerged from the plastic boxes of the first tape recorders that we had. At parties the lights were turned off whenever a blues was played and we danced in the dark kissing and fondling each other. Cigarettes and liquor circulated and encouraged us to defy the Comsomol taboos. Everything was now excitingly strange and forbidden. It was a privilege of a small elite group to enjoy the secret delights of these parties although there were always a few devious boys and girls with the right background and conventional manners who could get in by cheating.

My tiresome relation with literature reached an all-time low point with the appearance of a new teacher, Gencho Mollov. He was the archetypal dogmatic primitive Communist. On top of this he became my form master. His attitude to life was based on the Stalinist theory of class struggle and in his introductory speech to us he declared in Soviet textbook wording that there was most certainly a class enemy in our midst who eventually would be unmasked and crushed. I looked around me wondering who it could possibly be that he had in mind.

Mollov was a man of plain looks and humble peasant manners. His inbred hatred of civilisation which could be traced back to the primitive gloom of remote village life was his overwhelming characteristic. His profession offered him the opportunity to express his hatred since that was the one and only feeling characteristic of all literary works of Socialist realism that were mainly devoted to wild and rebellious villagers and tortured Soviet partisan women. Mollov was a man of great patience; he was ready to wait endlessly to identify the enemy and he quizzed us for our opinions with seeming naivety.

On one occasion on a school trip I wore a sweater with a tiny Swedish flag embroidered on the sleeve. Mollov could not fail to notice it. He approached me and asked me about my thoughts on West German revanchism. My doubts about its existence soon persuaded him that I was the exact class enemy that he sought.

I was immediately ordered to rip off the flag and severely reprimanded for misconduct. Mollov henceforward made a point of keeping a close watch on me so that he could assess exactly the degree of danger to the State represented by my survival. My essays on literature were subjected to the closest scrutiny and very soon they had persuaded him absolutely that I was the enemy in our midst.

I fell easy victim to Mollov's primitive analysis because in my youthful and intemperate way I lacked the cunning to keep my opinions to myself. I felt that things were taking a turn for the worse; it seemed to me that I was losing ground in my last year at school although in science and technology I was still far ahead of my classmates and indeed some of my teachers. I had the feeling that I was caught up in some absurd and desperate situation and my interest and motivation in doing well at school faded by the day.

On 3 November 1961 I was awakened at 5am by a group of strangers standing around my bed. I thought it was a bad dream but it all suddenly became painfully real.

A pair of plain clothes State Security agents had woken up my father and shown him a warrant for my arrest and for searching the house. My mother was out of town at a fashion show. My grandmother, brother and my sister also woke up because the four of us shared the bedroom. I got up and still dizzy with sleep, began to understand what was going on as one of the policemen escorted me to the toilet where he left open the door so that he could keep an eye on me.

The search ended with a written statement signed by Major Stoyan Taref, an inspector with State Security in the presence of my father and two neighbours called in as witnesses. The following objects all considered of interest to State Security were listed:

the text of an article I had sent to *Avto Moto*, a motor car magazine; the answer I had received from the editor; some letters from my Aunt Tanya in the USA and an obscure photograph whose subject I cannot remember.

I was taken in the patrol car to the central prison in Sofia and locked in a tiny cell in the basement after my belt and shoelaces had been removed.

I was not allowed to lie on my prison bunk after 5am and before nine at night but I sat on it to think about what had happened to me. Up to that time I had attracted the attention of the Secret Police on a few occasions; once as I made a casual remark in the street a plain clothes policeman suddenly appeared from nowhere, asked for my identity card and made a note of my name and address. But this was something quite different. As far as I knew it would not be easy to get out of a prison controlled by the State Security system. I felt wretched cooped up in this tiny cold cell with nothing in it but the bunk and a bucket surmounted by an oblong dish. Later I was informed that this was for carrying out my washing-up.

Soon Inspector Tarev obligingly gave me an explanation. He was a professional Stalinist interrogator; a man with deep experience in dealing with those very dangerous *enemies of the people* whom he happily sent off to the hellish existence of the detention camps. A classmate had been arrested some time previously after running away from home in what had been interpreted as an attempt to defect to the West. This young man frequently behaved like a clown during class breaks and could imitate Chaplin and Hitler in what I suspected to be a desperate attempt to attract attention. As a poor student he was unpopular and I felt sorry for him. His political parodies of Kruschev reminded me of the way Shego tried to compensate for his feelings of inferiority by inventing animals with disgusting habits; but these parodies were far more dangerous. Tarev explained to me that I was to be charged with establishing a political conspiracy; the so-called Congo Group that was supposedly aimed at toppling the present government. I was accused of plotting to form a new administration consisting of a selection of my seventeen year-old classmates headed by me taking over as Prime Minister.

Inspector Tarev was extremely serious about these charges. He had a copy of a plan of action for overthrowing the government in Sofia with a private army of two hundred men and he needed my confession to involvement in it. It occurred to me that he had probably succeeded in obtaining confessions to much graver charges from psychologically more stable adults and faced with a boy of seventeen his expertise in the various methods of persuasion would present no great difficulty. Within the walls of the State Security prison the concept of refusing to plead guilty did not exist. As interrogations continued it became obvious to me that Tarev shared Mollov's conviction that I was indeed an enemy of the State. I was accused of spreading bourgeois ideas among my fellow students; of being the sole perpetrator of numerous degenerate activities including rock and roll parties. It was really quite simple - there was always someone at the centre of each conspiracy who corrupted the others.

It seemed that it was the dream of every State Security police inspector to discover a conspiracy aimed at toppling the Government. I wondered what could have been the incriminating evidence against me that had been discovered at home. The article that they had found was concerned with the invention of a car body resistant to torsional loads and the magazine to which I sent it advised me in its reply to approach the Bulgarian Institute for Inventions. My Aunt Tanya's letters usually began with the conventional *My dearest and nearest* and would contain accounts of her family's regular moves throughout the United States. She wanted to invite my grandmother to spend time with her but that seemed impossible. During the period of my detention a dozen of my classmates were interrogated without result. It seemed that the only incriminating evidence available would be my own confession to the charges. The inspectors became desperate.

As I lay late at night shivering on my bunk and trying to sleep, an officer came to take me back to the interrogation room. It was about midnight and Tarev was accompanied by the four policemen who had arrested me that morning. There was a strong smell of wine in the air. As I was again asked about my plan to bring down the government with the aid of two hundred men two of the sturdy policemen removed their jackets and rolled up their sleeves. I realised what would happen and thought that only God could help me.

At that very moment the lights went out leaving us sitting in the dark. Because the power cut continued for some time the policemen became fed up and went home. I was taken back to my cell where some time later the electricity was restored and my naked light bulb glared at me throughout the night.

Perhaps it was not only irregular electricity supplies that prevented Tarev from consigning me to the notorious detention camp on the island of Belene in the Danube. Kruschev had already made considerable progress with his plan to dismantle the enormous machine of repression which formed the communist system and many of its victims had now been rehabilitated. Regrettably he was not allowed to finish the job and two years later was removed from power in an attempt to curtail his interference with the system. But in November 1961 it was Kruschev's ideas - the politics of the man who had recently exposed Stalin's crime at a Party congress - which directly prevented Tarev from proceeding with my interrogation. Kruschev, a man the Soviet Establishment if ever there was one, most probably saved my life.

Later I was informed that the father of a classmate had used his influence to apply Kruschev's philosophy to my advantage. He was probably able to give real assistance because of his position in the government machine. Tarev and his colleagues set me free but they would never forget or forgive me.

It was in fact the State Security department that governed the country because it controlled and intervened in all aspects of life. It maintained incriminating files on the population and thus had the destiny of all within its grasp. It was the State Security system that decided all aspects of punishment and imprisonment. In my case it was concluded that my personal convictions were anti-communist in nature and that I was without question intelligent. To demonstrate anti-ommunist thought within a group was considered to be extremely dangerous. Nevertheless the liberal tendencies of the period and my youth were found to be mitigating circumstances.

A parents' meeting was convened at my school and a high official of State Security described me as the driving force in a pro-Fascist group called Congo which had contaminated my classmates with bourgeois ideas. The school administration and the Comsomol Youth Organisation were ordered to decide my punishment. A dozen or so of my classmates were reprimanded for misconduct. In effect this meant that they would be forced to take their final examinations at a later date than their conformist fellows and would not be allowed to apply for admission to university before serving two years military service. Bobby was among these and was also expelled from Comsomol, thereby acquiring the status of a leper. I was excluded from all Bulgarian schools, denied the right to finish my secondary education and naturally expelled from the Comsomol. But while waiting for my punishments to be implemented I faced more trouble.

The world around me seemed to be falling apart and it was like an inescapable nightmare. I tried not to reveal my feelings to my family since they had already suffered enough. As though nothing had happened I continued to attend classes but I had an increasing sensation of a developing vacuum around me.

One December evening I went with a classmate to a fashionable café that had recently been opened opposite the park. Once called the Borisov Garden after the Czar, the park had a beautiful forest and long walks. It was snowing and the world seemed a pleasant place despite my problems. In the *Rusalka* café we observed a couple of

Those long school years

classmates and went to join them at their table. One of them liked to compete with me in physical strength.   He had already had a glass of brandy and imagined that his girlfriend fancied me. This seemed sufficient excuse to challenge me to fight him in the park.   However I did not take him seriously and left the café in the company of his friends.

These were all former students well known as outsiders and some were even petty criminals. They were certainly not friends of mine and some of them I met now for the first time.   Their leader was Dimiter Kalyashki, a hopelessly stupid student with an aggressive character. He was the nephew of a communist partisan killed in the wartime Resistance which had later secured for him the rank of an officer in the police force.

As we walked through the park my classmate soon calmed down and the conversation took a different turn. But he seemed uneasy about Kalyashki's friends following us along the snowbound alley.   One of them called out to me and as I turned round I received a heavy blow on the jaw. Caught unawares, I was probably standing with my mouth open when struck and my jawbone was broken in two places with one joint dislocated. I immediately fell down and as I staggered to my feet felt another blow in my face. I was unable to identify my attackers who by now were in the distance.

I spent a couple of months in hospital with my jaw in a splint. Each day my grandmother and mother brought liquid food. I now had all the time in the world for reflection. Beside this I had all the passion of an eighteen year-old. It transpired that the girl with whom I was in love was infatuated with the popular French screen idol Gérard Philipe. She was also hopelessly stupid and that helped me to get her out of my system.   While in hospital I spent hours making drawings of a small motor car on paper. The body was designed in a rather old-fashioned form and it had three seats. I also considered a new engine for it and this gradually took on an unconventional form. It resembled the chamber of a revolver but with pistons replacing the cartridges.

The only thing that I did not consider was my immediate future as I tried to put behind me the gloomy prospects lying ahead. I would be forced to join the army in the autumn and that seemed to represent the end of my world when the long school years would take an unfortunate and fatal, final turn.

I left hospital just as spring broke. I was now no longer officially a student and did not need to wear the obligatory dark blue uniform and cap. I returned to sit at my desk in my former classroom as I was summoned to attend a meeting of the local Comsomol branch at which my expulsion would be voted upon. My classmates realised that my future life was about to become very difficult and at the final vote the majority was against expelling me. It was painful to witness the overwhelming silence after the announcement of the vote followed by a raging torrent of abuse from the Comsomol functionary who was present to control the meeting. I stood up and declared that it was not necessary for him to put on a display since my convictions were definitely non-communist. I left the meeting. Some days later I was summoned to the City Committee of the Comsomol where another functionary explained to me in a friendly tone that the only philosophy which I could possibly embrace was the communist ideology. I was strongly advised to accept that if I wished to continue my studies. For the time being I would be subjected to a period of re-education during which I would work in a factory. The official said that he too had studied biology and understood my interest in science.

My father helped me finish my secondary education although that was strictly forbidden. He knew the headmaster of an adult education school who had no interest in the justification for my expulsion from school perhaps because so many of his students had been expelled, too, from some institution or other although perhaps not always for their political views. I applied to take the final examinations as a private student. Most of my fellow students were much older than I and among them were some policemen, one of whom grew to like me because I helped him pass his mathematics examination. I was also able to charm the literature teacher and was allowed to pass the examination although the subject was literature of the proletariat. Thus I finally succeeded in obtaining my certificate for secondary education and I even considered sitting the entrance exam for university where I wanted to study mechanical engineering. At the time all candidates had to be approved by a department of the city authorities and naturally my application was immediately turned down. An irritated official reminded me that I was supposed to work and not to apply for study at university.

The last summer of my school years began with a feeling of bitterness. As my classmates went to a ball in their first suits and party dresses I was left alone in the garden in the Congo corner where all my troubles had begun. I marked the occasion by making love to a girl for the first time in my life.

Chapter Three
Military Service

Most of my former classmates had already received call-up papers for military service and had left for barracks. When my papers finally arrived there was no indication of my destination. To judge by the railway station to which I was directed it appeared to be somewhere in the south.

During the summer I had tried to make the most of things. Affairs with girls and the short drive taken in the banana yellow Moskvitch car of a classmate were probably my most exciting moments. I was eager to make new friends but often switched from one to the other. A couple of girls took an interest in me but I was not attracted to them. The last days of my life as a civilian were spent wandering the streets in the hope of meeting my romantic ideal love.

Early one morning I arrived at Sofia central railway station with a dreadful haircut and carrying a small canvas bag containing a sandwich, razor and spare set of underwear. I left my mother and grandmother weeping among a crowd of distraught parents who had not been told where their children were to go. A sullen officer accompanied by a single soldier took charge of my group of ten young recruits. He pushed me on to the train to begin my two year period of military service.

I was seated in the compartment next to the escorting soldier. It was some time before he was prepared to tell me that we were headed for Kardzhali, a city near the border with Greece and Turkey. The other item of information that he divulged concerned the contents of the plain bag on his knees. This held our personal files and I realised that the miserable record of my short life for which I was going to pay during the years to come was right there in front of me barely fifty centimetres away. I was not allowed to read it.

To my group of newly arrived recruits in our prickly brown woollen uniforms everything seemed strange. Very soon reality was found to differ dramatically from my vague earlier ideas of army life. Personal hygiene was deplorable at the Kardzhali garrison. During the morning more than a hundred recruits were expected to wash with lightning speed at ten dribbling taps in a cold, narrow shed. Some of us did not even bother. The latrines were beyond belief. I had to muster all my resolve before I went to the toilet. The sweetest joy I could imagine would be the sight of the sergeant major stumbling and falling headfirst into the latrine.

During the winter, the windows of the hut where fifty of us slept were always tightly closed to retain the meagre warmth from a tiny coal-packed stove that showed a permanent reluctance to glow properly. At night the dormitory was suffused with the heavy, damp smell of footwrappings, those long cloth straps wound round their feet by soldiers instead of socks. Each stirring in bed raised clouds of dust and worked straw and twigs through the rough sackcloth pallets and pillows thrown on our bunk beds. The sheets were filthy and difficult to obtain since they made ideal replacement foot-cloths.

I quickly learned that it was essential for a soldier to carry all his possessions in his pockets. Anything left in the lockers at the end of each bed would promptly vanish. This meant that I had to carry with me my razor and a spoon; the latter for use when I found myself in the canteen with the opportunity to eat. There was never any cutlery provided there. I also had to carry all small personal objects including letters, photographs, a pencil and even a small device for cleaning rifles. Luxury was a spare set of underwear. According to the hygienic instructions in standing orders, shoes had to be polished before entering the canteen but there was no mention whatsoever of the need to wash our hands.

Nevertheless we ignored these minor problems, for as raw recruits we found ourselves living in a veritable nightmare. There was a well-established tradition in the Bulgarian army of subjecting recruits to permanent abuse by ordering them to carry out ridiculous orders that created a reign of physical and mental terror. Encouraged by the officers, this bullying often developed into acts of abuse and assault. Our principal tormentors were the junior NCOs who had been brutally trained for that very role. Second year soldiers in their turn maltreated raw recruits in order to take revenge for their own bullying and humiliation. This deep-seated hatred, violence and aggression towards raw recruits who had just joined the army passed like an infectious disease from one intake to the next, leaving deep scars in the minds of all on return to civilian life.

The military training that we were ordered to undergo was based on a series of tasks carried out in double-quick time and we were often bullied for fun by newly promoted superiors. We had to halt, return and carry out some stupid task over and over again until we nearly dropped with exhaustion. We were punished time after time for the slightest sign of rebellion and this would continue all day long and often well into the night. Having been brought to a state of virtual exhaustion, new recruits frequently suffered from insomnia interspersed with dreams of an elusive, precious moment of peace. But this insanity continued and finally progressed to cruelty until every man was reduced to dim-witted subhumanity, responding mechanically to the hysterically-screamed orders of the sergeant.

Some new recruits were forced to a state of total exhaustion. The growing hatred between superiors and the dominated assumed monstrous dimensions. Sometimes the reasons for this bullying were frankly absurd and we ten boys from Sofia were hated because we came from the capital. One among us - a weak and soft but well-educated boy with spectacles - was pushed around because his surname Kurodimov (*Cockdimov*) prompted obscene remarks and comments. It seemed that the humiliation of others was the only true source of satisfaction available to the sergeants and second-year recruits.

My own position was not particularly reassuring. Political rebels were unusual and my file had come to the notice of the officers. This was probably the first time that they had had to deal with such a creature. Among a hundred recruits there were only ten who had graduated from a high school and of these, only three, including me, wore spectacles. Because of my discreditable file, my task as an artilleryman was to be restricted to handing shells to the gunners. Like the other new recruits I was soon swept up in a whirlwind of being pushed around in a delicately balanced state between weariness and total exhaustion. Each morning when the sergeant inspected our dormitory, the scraps of sheet in which we had slept had to form a perfectly straight line which he would check with a long piece of string. One morning while straightening my sheets to meet the string I suddenly appreciated the appalling banality of the two years lying ahead of me.

At that time in autumn 1962 the chances of a third world war were greater than ever before. John F Kennedy, the US President, had wept when he realised that millions of

Military Service

Americans were at risk of death from nuclear attack by the Soviet Union. Having deployed nuclear missiles in Cuba the Russians were now sending ships to the island in defiance of an American blockade. The slightest violation would precipitate war and the entire military machine of the Eastern Bloc in a distant corner of which I now found myself as a raw recruit was preparing for this eventuality. Second-year recruits were retained beyond the normal demobilisation date and a section of the garrison was deployed in the mountains around Kardzhali.

As the first Soviet ship approached the blockading US fleet encircling Cuba, tension heightened. We observed that soldiers in our garrison were only occasionally ordered to carry out drill or checks on equipment and there was a dearth of reliable information about the international situation. Most of us had no idea of what was happening and no-one suspected that war could start at any moment. It is doubtful if we young recruits would have understood the position in any case.

The system created by Lenin was continuing to evolve and its strategic goal remained world supremacy. The lunatics at the top of the Soviet political hierarchy ached to achieve this goal in their own lifetime and many of them appeared ready to start a war if that was to be the price of success. The actual strategy for achieving world supremacy was however different. Western civilisation and the United States in particular would have to be forced to give in without a fight. This was described by the Kremlin as the policy of *peaceful coexistence*. At the same time Moscow unceasingly continued to attack the civilised world with all possible means short of nuclear war. This process was called the *ideological struggle*. Western civilisation was an impediment to the legitimisation of the Communist system and the destruction of capitalism was now to be given the highest priority.

Even Kruschev's determined efforts to liberalise the Soviet system failed to break down the formidable inbred dogmas of the Communist Party hierarchy. Attempts at reform were tolerated only so long as they could be employed in the struggle against western capitalism and at its heart, the United States. Any political movement, organisation or individual regardless of location would be given generous economic and military support if it were considered that they could damage the capitalist enemy. Fidel Castro was considered to be a great prize; he had made it possible to achieve the unthinkable: the deployment of nuclear missiles close to the shores of the United States where they could be used against American targets only minutes away.

Kennedy was quick to grasp the danger as he faced the choice between risking nuclear war and giving in to blackmail that could destroy his country without military conflict. That he chose to risk war and thereby forced Kruschev to surrender and withdraw Soviet missiles from Cuba is now distant history.

It was in fact more than a simple conflict between two strong men. Before long the popular Kennedy was assassinated and those behind his assassination ensured that his murderer Lee Harvey Oswald, who could have identified them, was in his turn done to death. Soon after that Kruschev - the one-time political commissar at Stalingrad now mouthing anti-Stalinist diatribes - was swept away. So too was the variety of maize seed which he had brought home from his visit to America to scatter on the vast steppes of the Soviet Union.

All these events took place during my two-year period of military service. At the exact time that the Soviet supply ships halted in the face of the American blockade of the Cuban approaches and Kruschev capitulated to Kennedy, I was enduring the worst period of my time as a raw recruit. Physical exhaustion and lack of sleep precluded my habitual peaceful thought and contemplation during the late evening hours. I was prepared to do anything if I could get a little sleep and relaxation and thought constantly of my family and friends whom I sorely missed.

One of my talents gave me a little comfort and respite from the endless hours of futile, exhausting activity. An artist was required, so I immediately offered my services and was assigned the task of painting heroic scenes, patriotic slogans and wall placards. I was much better at illustrations than text, and paint and other materials seemed either to be available in an extraordinary selection or not at all. I was prepared to use almost anything; green paint intended for anti-aircraft guns and other artillery requiring dilution in evil-smelling acetone thinners, or bright red poster paint delivered and applied in huge quantities. There was a permanent shortage of certain essential colours and often I would only have shaving brushes available with which to work, but judging by the reaction of my fellow soldiers, the results were not too bad.

My first painting appeared on the white wall at the end of the parade ground where each morning we lined up for drill. Its size was quite impressive; about ten metres long and two metres high. I drew an entire division in marching order and many of my fellow-soldiers scrutinized the work in an effort to detect resemblances between them and my heroic interpretation of the scene.

The winter of 1962 was severe in the extreme. The snow around Kardzhali was about a metre thick and the temperature at night dropped to minus ten degrees centigrade. Ammunition dumps in the surrounding mountains had to be guarded and each of us was sent up there at least once a week. The routine required standing for two hours on sentry duty followed by two hours in the guardroom on lookout and finally two hours asleep fully clothed; maintaining that shift rotation for twenty-four hours at a stretch. Standing guard at night between inner and outer barbed wire fences was unbearable but to fall asleep while on duty was considered a major offence punishable by transfer to special correction units in comparison with which normal military service routine was considered to be paradise.

I fought against the exhaustion and cold affecting my body and tried to imagine something to cheer me up a little. I began to think again about my engine and the small car to which it would be fitted in an effort to visualize what they would look like.

My parents and my grandmother came to Kardzhali a couple of times to see me. On the first occasion I felt a sharp pang when I realized the yawning gap between my world and theirs. They had to wait at the gates for me to finish my duty sweeping the dusty earth around the howitzers. Grandmother would visit me more frequently. She took a room in the city hotel where I could have a proper shower and eat the delicious food she brought with her on those occasions when I was allowed to take a few hours of leave. If not, she would stand at the gates talking to me and then depart. To visit me involved a train journey of more than eight hours.

Spring arrived and the cold days of winter faded into memory. My heavy wet boots and clothes dried out and life became a little more tolerable. The sinusitis that had dogged me all winter eased and a pleasant young lady doctor befriended me and arranged for me to stay and rest for two weeks at the local hospital. Hospital pyjamas and my shabby uniform made me feel awkward and I dared not flirt with her.

The summer brought further relief. I was less miserable about life at the garrison; comforting myself with the thought that soon I would only have a year of service left to do and the constant bullying by second-year recruits would perforce come to an end. The wonderful sunny weather and occasional moment of peace in a quiet corner of the barracks that it provided were really enjoyable after the extended nightmare of winter.

For summer duty my division was posted to the Black Sea coast near the northern border with Rumania. Near the small seaside town of Shabla there was a level cleared site with empty pillboxes and long-range artillery belonging to the coastal defence forces. There was a lighthouse nearby and a warm freshwater spring with the pungent smell of rotten eggs. We camped out in tents and carried out firing drill. The sea and sunshine made life almost pleasant and sometimes I would lie on my back on the dry hot earth and stare at the blue sky, lulled into a sense of infinite detachment accentuated by the distant thunder of anti-aircraft shellfire.

Autumn came and with it the great day of demobilisation dreamed of constantly by all second-year soldiers. A couple of days earlier one of them, a quiet and peaceful Pomak - as Muslims from the mountains around Kardzhali were called - visited me with a strange tale. He told me that on the very day that I had arrived he had been ordered by a Special Services officer (the military counterparts of State Security) to observe me and report everything that I did.

The Pomak was one of three soldiers in his draft who had been so instructed and he told me that one of them would always be on guard with me, ready to shoot me on the spot if I attempted to defect by heading for the border with my rifle as I was expected to do. I remembered that I was always on guard duty with one of the three. His sudden outpouring ended with the statement that he had always wanted to tell me about his orders because he was convinced that I was a decent fellow and to treat me that way was in his view, entirely wrong.

I was shocked by my own lack of awareness. Each one of those agents of the State Security service could easily have found an excuse to shoot me. They had not done so but who might follow them and fail to resist temptation? I never received an answer to that question but decided that in future it was essential that I should watch everything I said with the greatest care. This was not too difficult because I had only had close contact with a few of the Sofia boys in my group. If any of them had been an agent of the Security he could happily inform his superior of my ideas about inventing a four-stroke engine because I had openly talked about my plans.

After the new draft arrived in camp and I entered my second winter of military service, the time was approaching to choose my university course. It was clear to me that I would study mechanical engineering and more precisely follow the course dealing with internal combustion engines and automotive design. I wondered about a second choice since it was permitted to apply to two universities although passing the entrance examination did not automatically guarantee acceptance as a student. In order to successfully pursue further education I would need a favourable report on my background and career to date. That report would be issued by an employer or as in my case, by a commanding officer.

This report was handed to the prospective student in a sealed envelope and it was forbidden to read the contents. There were many applicants for university courses and for the arts faculty they completely outnumbered the places available. A law was passed allowing the children of elite communist *apparatchiks* with the status of *active fighters against capitalism* to enjoy special privileges and they would enter the university regardless of intellectual capacity. Parental connections, influence and conformity with the ideals of the State were of vital importance.

Near the end of the intricate maze that had to be negotiated to obtain a university place stood the political commissar, the second man in the chain issuing sealed envelopes. Mine - a colonel - was the fattest person in the garrison and his short stature made him look like a ball of moulded tallow. When we exercised he was particularly fond of calling out the pitch note for the Soviet Army marching songs in a melodious, high tenor voice.

Each day Bulgarian soldiers attended classes in political education. A combination of the conclusions to be drawn from our reaction to the humiliating training on the barrack square and behaviour in the classroom was intended to provide a judgement of our view of life. The advantages of socialism and the drawbacks of capitalism were the main subjects for discussion in such classes while the actual topics used were selected from the government-controlled daily press. Our officers were not gifted speakers and often asked me to repeat time and time again the drivelling party propaganda intended to awaken the drowsy audience. The service that I was thus able to provide gave me hope that the political commissar would be sympathetic and allow my application for university study to proceed without further delay.

To strengthen my position, my father had insisted that I should also apply for a course of study at his institute. As I sent in my application form immediately to him he was able to open in advance the sealed envelope containing the reference from the fat political commissar. My father therefore learned that the flabby musical colonel with the friendly smile had signed a report recommending that I should not be permitted to study in any university because of my unacceptable political views.

After my father warned me of the situation, I began feverishly to seek a solution. The commanding officer of my battery was a thin, inwardly withdrawn captain with a fondness for anisette. At the end of the day I knocked at his door, told him of my problem and asked for advice. He strode to the window, studied the dusty and deserted drill ground for some time and then spun round to tell me that I could write my own report and bring it to him for signature. He went on to admit that he had never wished to become an officer and that during his military service he had been trained as a reserve officer.   Then a government decree had arrived ordering all cadets to immediately take a regular commission to replace the former czarist officers who had been summarily dismissed.

In addition to automotive engineering I intended to study a fundamental scientific discipline. I imagined that there would be basic theories that extended to the extremes of human thought but I wished to peep beyond that. However, I did not believe in formal training in philosophy and decided to restrict myself to the study of engineering.

The short leave granted so that I could sit the entrance examinations seemed like a dream. I scored high marks and was among those at the top of the list to be admitted to study automotive engineering. Returning to the garrison to complete my military service depressed me and I methodically counted the days to my formal discharge.

During this period my grandmother was allowed to visit her daughter Aunt Tanya who had finally settled in California after following a nomadic existence for fifteen years. The news of Grandmother's visit to the United States was breathtaking and she came to visit me in order to say goodbye. She was now sixty-two and bursting with energy and courage. I was the most important person in her life and we spent

Military Service

time discussing our plans for the future. She wanted me to visit her in the United States but that seemed out of the question and we carefully avoided any further mention of it. She was terrified by the idea that I might attempt to defect and made me swear that I would not take such a risk. At that time there was absolutely no possibility that I would receive permission to travel abroad although she believed that there might be some way in which I could officially leave the country because so many things that once seemed impossible had been successfully achieved in recent years. We bade each other farewell at the garrison gate and my grandmother left bearing my thoughts and fantasies about the unknown and exciting California.

My last months in the army were a combination of ill-tempered impatience and a series of attempts to plan my future. I considered the engine and car that I would one day build but I could not imagine what my life would be like in the years to come although I knew that the world outside was changing rapidly. One evening at the end of that summer the music of an American pop song blared out from the loudspeakers and prompted the special services officer to ask me whether my grandmother could send him material for a suit from the United States. Kruschev had vanished but the Iron Curtain was already torn and admitting the wind of change. Things would never be the same again.

Finally my demobilisation papers arrived and feeling awkward in my civilian clothes of two years ago, I walked through the gates leaving behind me the plywood wall that I had once decorated. This was one of the happiest days of my life. The train slowly drew out of Kardzhali, transporting me in a state of youthful euphoria towards the mirage of a future of infinite beauty.

Chapter Four
What will I be when I grow up?

The Lenin Higher Mechanical and Electrotechnical Institute was situated in the barracks of the one-time garrison of Ministry of the Interior forces established to protect communism from its internal enemies during the 1950s. The buildings were characteristic of that period; ugly blocks with the small windows and massive pillars typical of Stalinist architecture, erected in an open field near Sofia. This area was known as Darvenitsa (bedbug) and later when converted into a huge housing estate it was renamed Mladost (youth). In front of the former barracks buildings trapezoid-shaped halls had been constructed on wide straddling supports. Long corridors connected the barracks to the halls. The surrounding barren countryside was either muddy or dusty according to season and it took us students over an hour to reach the Institute in one of the overcrowded buses emitting foul-smelling diesel fumes.

I found myself one among what appeared to be thousands of students coursing through the endless corridors. Lectures were attended by hundreds of students in large auditoria and our working groups contained thirty or forty boys and girls in each of the smaller classrooms. Our curriculum was very intensive and we took classes from early morning untl late in the afternoon. Because there were so many students there was little room left for individual contact with lecturers and the prospect of wasting an hour on the bus ride made me eager to leave that dismal windy open place as soon as my classes were at an end.

My personal comfort at home had improved. My grandmother's absence in the United States and my brother's military service meant that I only had to share the room with my sister. I converted the small attic room on the sixth floor so that I could study. It was only two by four metres and had a small window and a door which opened on to a narrow corridor. This room was furnished with an old wooden bed, a broken-down table and two chairs on their last legs. Although it was always dusty this attic was a dream indeed for a student at that period.

My friend Bobby had been admitted to study construction engineering and was lucky to have his institute only a ten-minute walk from the city centre. Shego studied there too; he had succeeded in entering the Institute immediately after completing his study at the high school. He would now do his military service after graduation or at any time might drop out; the chances of that were steadily increasing with the passage of time.

There was now a new café opposite the city garden not far from the Congo corner and the American embassy. It was named Rosa and Shego was a regular customer, spending all his time there in the company of fellow students. Their main occupation seemed to be mocking and sneering at each other and Shego was right in the middle of this - as before, enthusiastically composing love poems and inventing fictional amorous escapades.

Bobby introduced me to Dimitar (Mitko) Penev, a friend from his army days. Mitko studied medicine and was the most brilliant student of his year. He was tall with a long slender neck and a smiling narrow face with thick spectacles. Despite this he was in fact a surprisingly strong and successful athlete. But it was his intellect that fascinated me most.

With great ease he read widely beyond the compulsory set books on anatomy and physiology. In pursuit of his own personal curriculum he studied physics, mathematics and scientific philosophy; devouring dozens of books on these subjects simultaneously.

Soon Mitko and I became the best of friends. We exchanged books on every subject; on philosophy and logic as well as biology and cybernetics. In our shared study of recently published articles we discovered the genetics and computer sciences that had long been rejected as bourgeois nonsense. We discussed various subjects but concentrated our attention on two philosophical problems; those aspects in which living organisms differed from inanimate matter, the essence of genetic information and the origins of life.

I was excited by this new world opening to me after the long spiritual isolation of my army life. I read Camus and Kafka which were available published in limited editions. I introduced Shego's rebellious friends to those of Mitko and Bobbie at the Rosa café where I indulged myself by attracting attention with my fictional stories. But gradually my interest in idle discussion and wild partying at the café waned. It was only my friendship with Mitko that endured as we continued our discussions with vigour.

I was eager to meet new people and longed for the stimulus of interesting minds. I seriously sought an ideal girlfriend who could satisfy the longing of my heart. Not one of the girls among the hundred first-year students in my faculty who arrived sleepily each morning to attend the lectures in the large halls even approached my ideal. I realised that I had failed to establish meaningful contact with my fellow students.

The subjects that I studied at the Institute were of a general nature and had little association with cars. Soon I discovered that I was exceptionally good at all those subjects requiring imagination in three dimensions such as geometry and drawing. I could easily visualize surfaces and shapes and was quick to pinpoint their intersecting lines and projections without the use of formal methods. My innate abilities impressed the assistant lecturer and I was exempted from the examination. But in other subjects I had great difficulties as a result of my total lack of formal memory. I could easily handle formulae and algorithms if I had a reference book at my disposal; but as soon as I turned the page I forgot everything. As books of reference were banned from examinations and huge amounts of data had to be memorized, my results were generally poor.

It was during that autumn that the natural evolution of my invention persuaded me to take the first step towards the profession that I would follow some thirty years later. I had devised an automatic gearbox. Applied to an inclined plane surface, the power of the engine was channelled into two directions; one of which was devoted to the automatic changing of gear. It was the same concept that later brought me success but at that time I was making impatient attempts to apply it to a mechanism of unusual construction but distinct technical naivety. Whether my idea was convincing or not I determined to launch it and filed for an *author's certificate*; the Socialist counterpart of a patent at the Bulgarian Institute of Inventions.

Naturally my automatic gearbox was doomed to failure once it had been subjected to proper analysis. I had stumbled upon the idea and did not attach much importance to it. To my mind an automatic gearbox was nothing but a clever solution achieved via a simple mechanism. I was twenty-one and eager to try my hand at more important matters before I could determine my future. The failure therefore meant little to me and I continued to think about cars and their mechanisms in a light-hearted manner with no firm goal in mind. I was not sure at this time what I wanted to do in the future and would have been surprised indeed if anyone had forecast a successful life based on my work on automatic transmissions.

What will I be when I grow up?

My parents had limited means and were hardly able to pay for the education of their three children. We still shared our flat with other tenants. If there was to be a real ray of hope it was not to arise from my filing a patent but more from Grandmother Stoena's activities in California. Soon after the excitement of her arrival in California had subsided my grandmother and Aunt Tanya established a day nursery and shared the profits. Characteristically Grandmother put by every dollar that she earned and soon her savings amounted to a real fortune in our eyes. She often wrote in her spidery hand, describing with many misspelt, colourful expressions how much she missed and loved us. Sometimes she would send me a small gift of dollar bills.

Spring arrived and again I longed for the holidays when the weather would be sunny and warm and life beautiful. A few examinations remained and I had to follow a training course; none of which afforded much inspiration. I was posted as a trainee to an electric truck plant where I found little inspiration for my future profession. One morning after arriving in the ancient fume-filled machine shop where in appalling dust and noise the workers were hammering the slag off welds on a rough chassis I suddenly realised that this was not in the least a career for me. But how could I find my way to California? At that time it seemed the most impossible thing in life and this was absolutely so.

My grandmother needed a document that had to be validated at the American embassy. I went there and handed it to a very polite secretary. Next week I was summoned to appear at the local
police station where an officer with a florid complexion interrogated me on every detail of my two-minute visit to the embassy. Slowly and clumsily completing his notes on the papers lying over his desk he asked me again why I had visited the American embassy. I did my best to keep calm but felt that it hardly mattered and indeed he needed no excuse to start shouting at me and threatening me by saying that I was not to go there any more unless I wanted to have trouble with him. It was obvious to me that to leave for the United States was quite out of the question.

Shortly before the summer holidays I met a tall slim girl with peroxide blonde hair and blueish-grey eyes. It was a mutual interest in Hemingway's books that brought us together and she agreed to go out with me. Her name was Vera and she claimed that she was a student at the Fine Arts Academy. With her fashionable hairdo, tight short dress and high heels she drew the attention of all even when walking on the other side of the street and I did not mind that at all. Bobby thought her nose somewhat long but all my friends agreed she was quite pretty. Soon we met every evening and she accepted my invitation to spend the holidays with me at the seaside.

We went to Galata, a small village on the Black Sea, south of Varna where a schoolfriend of mine lived. We rented a room on a farm and spent our days on the beach and our evenings in the village pub in the company of my friend. We had a lovely time but I felt that inside Vera hid a shy hesitant little girl tormented by complexes and innumerable problems beyond solution. It transpired that I was correct and after the short holiday our relationship seemed overwhelmed by absurd discussion as Vera sank ever deeper into her inner discomfort. Often in the evening after walking with her under the trees in the beautiful small streets near the Alexander Nevski cathedral I went home with a feeling of profound relief and spent hours reading a book or drawing the car of my dreams.

Bobby remained my best friend and we continued our discussions just as we had at school. He fell in love with a married woman he met at the seaside - she was about thirty years old; a short thin and intelligent woman. Her husband regularly drank himself into a stupor and discussed the absurdity of life with Bobby. She still lived with him and their six year-old daughter although their relationship had been hopelessly damaged. Desperately in love with her, Bobby himself took to heavy drinking and gave in to his irrational destructive moods. By the end of the summer and during the autumn Bobby and his girlfriend became gradually overcome by a combination of inner despair, decadence and alcohol. Vera felt ill at ease with them and grew yet more depressed. Branimir, who had just completed his three years of military service and was now obsessed with a feeling of total absurdity, soon joined our group. While waiting for his draft notice, Shego, who had failed in his studies, shared with us his comic sentimentality and pages of unreadable poetry. In his darker moods Bobby would be drunk for days on end. Soon my relationship with Vera reached a low point and I engaged in much inner torment before I was able to break with her. Bobby, who was up to his ears in the mire of his own love affair, shared my problems. He too felt ready to go to extremes because of his feelings - in fact he did many stupid things including giving up studying and taking a job at a paper factory working in a three-shift system.

I wrote a short story in which I tried to assemble all the elements of my experience. In the end the hero of my tale jumped on to his motorcycle and sped off. However I had nowhere to go and the text did not inspire me to continue writing. I had no aspirations to become a writer but I had lost interest in engineering and could hardly imagine how I would make a living.

Mitko was the only one among us who avoided trouble. He was devoted to science and worked extremely hard, at the same time abstaining from drinking alcohol and smoking while keeping a smiling face. We met regularly and our discussions deepened. Because he was an insatiable reader I was able to take advantage of his summaries which saved me from reading piles of paper. On the other hand I was the more creative in the interpretation of these facts and Mitko in turn appreciated that. Gradually we discovered the imperfection of certain established theories like Darwin's *The Origin of Species* and found ourselves confronted by a lack of fundamental explanations of biological phenomena. It was that scientific journey that brought me ever nearer to physics.

One day Mitko lent me Einstein's little book on the special and general theory of relativity. I simply devoured it and was thrilled by the beauty of this creation of the human intellect. Simultaneously I was fascinated by this new field of human thought which immediately attracted me with the vast opportunities it allowed for imagination and research. I felt a strong desire to become a physicist. Whatever I did, my thinking had already begun to operate to its own full satisfaction in this new, recently discovered world.

Besides encountering Einstein's theory through Mitko, I met some of his friends who came together to discuss philosophical subjects. Most of them were students of philosophy, philology or physics who had a natural liking for abstract, highbrow discussion. Their style was somewhat academic and dry compared to Bobby's smoky and liquor-drenched parties. I joined in those discussions but felt myself somewhat out of place. The high-flown scholastic atmosphere was set by a philosopher among them who had assimilated Marxist doctrines and the work of Hegel from the official discourses taught at the university. Sometimes I was tempted to interject one of Shego's filthy words commonly used by my own friends.

During the winter I realised that I had to make up my mind about what I wanted to do. My own way of thinking was very different from the methods used at the Institute; there was a yawning gap between the new physics that attracted me with its ideas and the established physics that I was taught in class. To pass our examination we were forced to learn by heart thousands of short formulae with little or no practical purpose. It was not difficult for me to manage the theory of physics and the basic engineering sciences, but I was not at my best in the matter of committing pages of factual material to memory. Besides this I no longer felt myself to be motivated to become involved in that type of competitiveness. The workload was heavy, the curriculum detailed and extensive and students were expected to work extremely hard during long days, showing the sort of diligence and application one would expect in a secondary school. Besides this, the long hours spent on the bus travelling from the city centre to the Institute to attend lectures that were frankly a disappointment was for me a total waste of time. It was essential for me to look for more suitable conditions if I were to continue to develop my own process of contemplative thought.

The Academy of Fine Arts had introduced a course in industrial design and this caught my attention. It suggested the combination of my passion for motorcars with art and was probably a good environment for me in which to indulge my scientific hobbies. I was an accomplished artist and the Academy of Fine Arts was an elitist institution because of its access to and connections with the relaxed life of the artists' community, much favoured by the authorities. As soon as I heard of this course in industrial design I resolved to attend it. This however was a rather presumptuous decision; admission to the Academy was difficult to say the least, with more than two hundred applicants for every place, but I was confident that I would succeed in becoming one of the lucky ones.

In the meantime my grandmother had returned from California armed with several thousand dollars that she had saved. This made her extremely important in our society where the possession of foreign hard currency was one of the most desirable virtues of the time because of the opportunity and right that it gave to the holder to buy Western consumer goods including motor cars in the special *Corecom* shops. The goods available on the market were of uniformly bad quality and the few models of East European cars available in Bulgaria required a long wait sometimes even more than twenty years, with prior payment terms.

My grandmother was extremely happy to be back with us and looked very well. She planned to visit America again and was now my comfort and support at home as my father became increasingly unsure and nervous about my plan to switch my course of studies. Most importantly, she wanted to buy a car for me; something that could make my sweetest dreams come true. My father hesitated but eventually agreed and we chose a white four-door Ford 12M that could be delivered to us within a matter of a couple of months.

The return of my grandmother made me sad because in my search for a future profession I had not come any nearer to my original Californian dream. I came to the realisation that whatever it was that I wanted to do I would always be faced with the same basic problem: when and how could I leave Bulgaria? At the moment the only prospect seemed to be to defect. I was still a young man but the clock inside me kept ticking away to remind me of the time that I was wasting, and had a very unsettling effect on me.

I sat for the industrial design entrance examinations without any preparation. The examination required an academic pencil portrait, a sculptured copy of an antique bust and a scale model of a water tap. In the throng of applicants a slim girl with freckles and green eyes impressed me with her artistic manners. Her name was Rositsa. I asked her if she would like to be my friend and she said that she was sorry but she was hopelessly involved already with a boyfriend. This was the first time that a real girl offered something of the fictional world that impressed me so much. But just as it always was in my favourite books, everything seemed lost and doomed from the outset. There was only a feeling of deep irrational understanding between us and the whole affair ended with a couple of brandies in a nearby café. Rositsa was bound to fail the examinations but I found that I was among the first to be admitted.

I felt very lonely in my relationship with girls. A year previously during an autumn evening, Shego's great love Nina - to whom he had consistently dedicated his love poems since the lower classes of the high school - suddenly asked me to take her home after a party. She confessed that she had loved me secretly for years and was ready to do anything I asked. I was more than surprised since I had noticed nothing of this at all. Nina said that I failed to notice most of the things going on around me and claimed that she had never been on intimate terms with Shego or anyone else as she had already decided that I was to be the first man in her life. This made me feel extremely awkward. I tried to be friendly and to convince her that she had no chance of winning my heart, but Nina insisted that she already knew that and had accepted it long ago. Since then we occasionally went out together but I took every opportunity to demonstrate that I did not care for her. Nevertheless, deep inside me I felt lonelier after those times together.

The Academy of Fine Arts was situated in the centre of Sofia behind the Alexander Nevski cathedral. The industrial design studios occupied a late nineteenth century two-storey house near the university. It faced the National Library and a small park known as the Doctors' Garden because it contained a small memorial to medical personnel killed in the War of Liberation. At the time I was unaware that this would be one of the most beautiful places in my experience but I was always happy to be there.

I had six fellow students in my group, all boys. One of them Rusi Dundakov, soon became my good friend. He was a good-looking athletic boy with a volatile temperament with moods fluctuating from glowering rage to charming good humour and he would pass through this range in an artistic manner. At first he watched me quietly from a distance and then came to introduce himself with a sour expression but quickly told me in an animated and interesting way about his last days of army service.

I already knew another of my fellow students. Dimitar Milev was the notorious founder of the first Bulgarian pop group, *The Bandaratsite*; local rivals to the Beatles. He was universally known as Bandaraka and many were totally unaware of his real name. He was short and so thin that he appeared emaciated, had thick dark curly hair rather too long for a good Communist with rectangular-framed spectacles and blue jeans. He was somewhat eccentric and very unusual. As a born artist he had a rebellious charm and disregard of convention. He drank to excess and sometimes created extremely embarrassing situations but we all nevertheless liked him well and never lost our temper with him.

Part of the curriculum included the academic drawing of models, human anatomy and the history of art. We students of fine arts and those of the applied arts department were required to attend all these classes in addition to a series of lectures on technique. Unfortunately our industrial design lecturer was far from satisfactory and not au fait with modern practice. It was he who had established the course but there was in fact little he could teach his students and he and I were soon on openly hostile terms. Despite all this, the general atmosphere and our activities were like paradise compared with those inflicted on us at the Engineering Institute.

Then I appeared with a new white Ford car in our street. The automobile that I had always carried in my being like a magic idea had finally emerged in the shape of that very

What will I be when I grow up? 53

car and I was now beside myself with excitement and joy. There were very few cars on the streets of Sofia and it was easy for me to park the Ford between two Moskvitch that remained motionless for most of the time. I was the only one in our family to hold a driving licence.

Sometimes I would take the entire family with me for a drive into the countryside. In actual fact we could not afford to run the car. My brother was studying at my father's institute, my sister was in the first year in the high school; we had used up my grandmother's savings from America and we still had to find the rent for our flat. In the following year we sold the car and with the proceeds were able to buy the flat as our joint tenants moved out after twenty years of cohabitation. Grandmother immediately left for America again although she was already sixty-six years old. On this occasion she was absolutely determined to buy a car that would be for me alone. I asked myself: would that still be in Sofia?

During the past year the desire to create my own vehicle had concentrated on a motorcycle design project. I had become rather bored by the soporific although easygoing and pleasant routine at the Academy and now looked for a proper design project to pursue. In the spring a fellow student and I went to the Applied Design Centre recently established to serve heavily bureaucratic Bulgarian industry. We offered our services as volunteers in exchange for the opportunity to get experience in our future profession. Our offer was gladly accepted and we were put to work with clay on a design project for a motorcycle intended for Bulgarian mass production. One day at a manufacturers' meeting our improvised models were presented next to the official proposal - we assumed that the Design Centre organisers were anxious to give the impression of bustling activity. The manufacturers liked our models and we were invited to compete with the Design Centre in the final round when the future model for motorcycle production would be selected.

The idea fascinated us. I established an open air studio on the roof of the apartment house which had a large terrace surrounded by numerous chimneys and small sheds where we would play cards. There my fellow student and I made two plaster casts of a motorcycle, painted them and presented them to the selection committee. My model was clear favourite but naturally the administrative machine that automatically disapproved of my personal behaviour opted for the crude model submitted by the Design Centre itself. The new motorcycle based on that design was so ugly that it failed to attract buyers and production was soon brought to an end.

In the autumn I decided that it was now time for me to begin all over again to make a determined effort to defect to the West.

I had no idea how I would earn my living abroad but I knew for certain that there would be no future for me in Bulgaria.

In 1967 there was no chance that I would receive a passport allowing me to travel abroad. Kruschev's brave détente had been smothered by the old regime in Moscow led by Brezhnev. The new hardliners tried to restore the gaps in the Iron Curtain as they realised that infiltration by Western ideas would threaten their own repressive system. The reformist movement in Czechoslovakia was also smothered at that time and there was a general further tightening of all the regimes and political police in the Eastern bloc. With no alternative, thousands in all the repressed Communist countries now dreamed of defecting to the West and were prepared to sacrifice everything to realise their dream.

In Bulgaria, Zhivkov maintained his tight grip on the regime having built his career on the brutal repression in Sofia of the 1940s. In every sphere he maintained a policy of closest possible cooperation and dedication to the Soviet leadership. His once widely advertised fondness for Kruschev did not prevent him from now demonstrating an even greater loyalty to the arch-conservative Brezhnev. At the beginning of the 1970s he surpassed himself by suggesting to the Soviet Union that it should annex Bulgaria but thankfully his plan did not fit Soviet foreign policy and was never realised. Nevertheless Bulgaria was virtually an integral part of the Soviet Union in all respects.

Zhivkov was cast in the standard mould of all primitive communist dictators and controlled everything that went on in Bulgaria including what films should be shown, what hairstyles worn and even on the local appointment of managers in small industrial enterprises. Despite his ludicrous manners and appearance he had an exceptionally vindictive and accurate memory - the Bulgarian writer Georgi Markov was assassinated in London after publishing a selection of pointed and accurate comments on his contacts with Zhivkov. The famous Bulgarian umbrella assassination technique was used on this occasion to kill Markov with a poison dart. Zhivkov's daughter was fawned on by the authorities and was allowed to spend millions on crazy pseudo-cultural projects. Zhivkov had converted the village of his birth into a prosperous town and built a motorway to connect it to Sofia. Literary works officially written by him were published in exclusive editions and translated into a plethora of foreign languages; his speeches were regularly quoted and his ugly portrait displayed widely in all public places.

A strongly repressive organisation maintained Bulgaria's isolation from all other countries and excluded foreign influences while at the same time repressing all opposition and deviation from the official party line. In 1966 a special department of State Security was inaugurated - the so-called Sixth Department - intended to combat all *ideological sabotage*. This was to include any deed, statement or thought that clashed with the official policy maintained by hordes of policemen with unlimited power and highly sophisticated electronic bugging equipment. These in turn were supported by hundreds of thousands of official informers and many amateurs who were happy to report on their fellow citizens. This apparatus spied on and bugged all those suspected of subversive activity and could easily maintain watch on the entire population. Policemen working with the Sixth Department - the so-called operational officers - enjoyed unrestricted access to all and were able to interfere in every institution since all those in the organisation from the workshop management up to the chief executive were obliged to report to them.

Over one million of the total population of eight million Bulgarians were members of the Communist Party. The important functions and tasks were reserved for Party members who had been carefully screened and approved. In the scramble for privilege and career opportunities many citizens were prepared to do anything that would demonstrate their political reliability. This resulted in a stifling and corrosive atmosphere throughout the country. The highly inefficient manufacturing industry was descending into chaos and maintained only by bolstering with foreign loans. Most people were resigned to the situation and passively accepted the levelling of wages, lack of incentives and total dependence on the state administration. Press, radio and television were all state-controlled. Writers, artists, actors and film producers competed in their efforts to praise Zhivkov and his regime. Scientific centres and universities took every precaution not to develop an idea that might be construed as opposition to established communist dogma. All information, all cultural and artistic influences from abroad was censored and admitted only if it could demonstrate how capitalism was doomed and rotten. Travel abroad was only allowed to those considered to be entirely trustworthy.

What will I be when I grow up?

Again it was the State Security system that controlled travel abroad and dealt with unsuccessful defectors. The law handed down five years imprisonment for those who attempted to defect and those who helped them. During that period about one hundred and fifty people succeeded in escaping from Bulgaria each year and about the same number failed to return from officially permitted travel abroad. More than four hundred were shot dead at the heavily guarded borders; particularly after security was strengthened in the 1970s. Frequently East Germans would attempt to defect via Bulgaria and many were caught or shot in the act.

During the 1960s it was usually via Yugoslavia that East Europeans tried to escape to the West. Citizens of communist countries were allowed to travel in the Eastern bloc without a special passport - just with a simple permit that was usually issued without question. That permit would allow the holder to travel via Yugoslavia to another Eastern European country and the Yugoslavian border with Italy and Austria was not particularly heavily guarded and was therefore easier to cross allowing many to successfully flee. Yugoslavia had an official agreement with Bulgaria to return all defectors but the authorities were generally more liberal and Yugoslavian citizens themselves were free to travel wherever they wished.

Some of my former classmates had succeeded in escaping via that route; one returned after a failed attempt and gave me some helpful information. Unfortunately it turned out to be somewhat inaccurate and I assumed that he was in fact afraid to tell me all the details. As part of my escape plan I applied for a permit to travel to Prague. In October 1967 I boarded the night train with a small sum of money and a suitcase. Nina came to bid me farewell at the station and she was the only one who knew of my intention. In the morning I arrived in Belgrade and bought a ticket to Zagreb where I spent the night walking round and waiting for the train to Ljubljana. My precautions appeared unnecessary for no-one asked for my passport and I was able to buy a ticket to any destination I chose. The last of my money was spent on buying a ticket from Ljubljana to Sezhana on the Italian border, ten kilometres from Trieste. According to my advice I was to arrive late at night so that I could attempt to cross the border on foot under cover of darkness.

The train arrived in Sezhana just before midnight and I got out on to the small platform. The Slovenian tongue spoken in that area was different and incomprehensible to me unlike the Serbo-Croatian which I could easily understand thanks to its similarity to Bulgarian. It was because of this that I was unable to obtain information from the few passengers who left the train and vanished into the deserted streets of Sezhana. With a suspect sense of direction I walked down the main street and soon came to the outskirts where I decided that it was logical to set out towards the hills that rose indistinctly in the dark on my right.

The night was silent and the weather mild but there was no moon and after a few hundred metres I found myself walking in total darkness. Occasionally headlights from distant cars would give me an idea of the topography. Eventually I climbed a hill at the foot of which were terraced fields separated by stone walls each about a metre high. As I climbed towards the top I found myself bumping into ever-thicker thorny shrubs which caught at the hem of my raincoat. Moreover the ground was damp and clumps of mud accumulated on the thin soles of my shoes as I stumbled over the boulders in my path.

After wasting over an hour on my difficult climb I realised that I had walked barely five hundred metres without nearing the summit. I decided to change direction and despite the huge amount of energy that I wasted during the following hours considered that I had hardly covered more than a kilometre and was still no nearer the border. I stopped to rest and by the light of a match saw that I was in a dreadful state. My raincoat was torn and covered in mud;

my shoes, socks and trousers were thick with mud and my hands lacerated. It was almost five o'clock which meant that I had been wandering for over four hours. I had no money left and it was clear that my plan was doomed. In order to avoid being caught in that state I must leave for Bulgaria on the first available train although I had no ticket. I was ignored at the Bulgarian border despite having no raincoat. Only my mother expressed concern and during the night when I had been in Sezhana she had dreamed a nightmare in which I struggled agonizingly through undergrowth and mud.

Ten days later I applied again for a new permit to the same destination. The Bulgarian regulations stipulated that only one permit per annum would be allowed to each citizen but this appeared to be disregarded and I quickly received my new permit. I tried to obtain more advice from the boy who claimed to have crossed the border at Sezhana. I then saved up some money and bought a pair of stronger shoes and in November set out again on the same journey; finding myself at midnight again on the railway platform in Sezhana.

This time the night was clear and the cloudless sky was lit by a half-moon. According to the information in my possession I had to follow the right-hand side of the road that led from the main street until I arrived close to the checkpoint. I would then have to circle to the right. I walked a hundred metres along the road so that I would not be observed by passing cars and again came to the terraces at the foot of the hill. I then returned to the road and crossed three kilometres of rugged terrain before spotting a lighted building that was probably the checkpoint. I climbed the hill to avoid the road and then walked as far as I could and headed west in the direction where I imagined Trieste to lie. After a while it seemed to me that I was descending and thought that I saw lights and heard the noises of a town. I wondered whether I had already crossed the border and felt like running towards my unknown future in the free world ahead.

I emerged into an open space that looked like a clearing among the trees. I did not like the idea of being spotted so I strode across as quickly as possible. Just before I reached the security of the trees again, a soldier armed with a machine gun sprang up in front of me and shouted words that I could not understand. He continued to shout in a way which indicated that I had to drop something until I realized that he meant the bag that I carried in my hand. I was then taken to the checkpoint and the soldiers searched my luggage and checked my papers. Their superior, a sergeant somewhat younger than I, said that they were sorry that they had caught me and would not have done so if they had realized that I was Bulgarian. They appreciated that once back home I would be sent to prison. Soon two policemen arrived and took me to the police station in Snezhana.

In the morning the policeman who had interrogated me and had prepared a written statement delivered me to the railway station and put me on the train back to the Bulgarian border. He seemed friendly, offered me a cup of coffee and tried to comfort me by assuring me that there could possibly be no adverse consequences of my attempted defection. I was so tired that I fell immediately asleep as soon as I sat in the train. When I was awakened to change trains I began to realize what had happened and felt that at that point in my life I could not even begin to understand what lay ahead for me.

Chapter Five
Profession and Hobby

Hardly anyone at the Academy of Fine Arts noticed that I had missed a number of classes. I had expected to be interrogated by officers from State Security but no-one checked up on me. By the end of the autumn I had reached the conclusion that the Yugoslavian authorities had not sent an official report of my detention at the border to their counterparts in Bulgaria.

It was not possible for me to take seriously the way in which industrial design was taught at the Academy but at least it was not a difficult or tedious subject. Our lecturers rushed through their classes and seemed to have no real interest in the subject of design. Most of the time we were left alone with the six of us standing around a lump of clay or an easel engaged in futile discussion.

Rusi and I were close friends. He enjoyed making up stories crammed with exotic imaginings and his descriptions of people and events were richly embroidered with his own fantastic thoughts. He followed a hardly rational logic of his own which nevertheless was somewhat convincing. He was easily provoked to anger and his rage could be destructive, but he was also a charismatic character and had a splendid sense of humour. We had both read Hasek's *Svejk* and often referred to passages that we had committed to memory.

Rusi was narcissistic and egocentric in behaviour and was a good mixer with all sorts of people. Most of his circle were artists and actors and I tried to keep up with their personal style. Rusi was a heavy drinker but also a gifted entertainer. He was an excellent guitarist and sang Russian and gypsy songs with great skill. He gave me the nickname of *Horse* and provided me with fanciful roles in his whimsical tales.

At the annual ball of the Academy one of the first-year students, a beautiful girl with long blonde hair, showed open interest in me. Her name was Krasimira but she insisted on being called Mariana. Rusi nicknamed her the *Tyrolese* because of the short Tyrolean skirts she liked to wear. Beauty compensated somewhat for her boring nature but her incessant jabbering often reduced me to despair and I quietly wished that I could disappear at the first opportunity. Soon I was able to turn a deaf ear to her while apparently maintaining my interest. This was not particularly difficult as I had virtually nothing to say in return and it enabled us to achieve a certain harmony.

Bobby left for Moscow to continue his study of geology begun a year earlier. His love affair had ended in increasing agony. Soon after arriving in Moscow he met a Bulgarian student and quickly became engaged to her. That made me sad and the moment that I saw his fiancée when she returned to Sofia for the wedding I wondered what it was that could keep them together. The future that Bobby and I had dreamed of for years began to appear very different.

Shego too was now married. After military service he returned to his studies; this time at my father's institute. His passion for poetry intensified and he collected together and bound his work in volumes. His chosen girlfriend, a nondescript student from the provinces, was interested neither in poetry nor in his circle of friends but she soon became pregnant and they were obliged to marry.

Third in the row was my own brother who became involved with a fellow student from the country; a pretty girl who fairly rapidly became pregnant and reduced his freedom of manoeuvre. He moved into her parents' flat in the Sofia suburbs and once again I was able to enjoy some privacy in our apartment where I continued to live with my parents and sister. Of course I still had my tiny attic room, too.

Mitko continued to make progress with his medical studies and we continued our theoretical discussions. He resisted the temptation of the artistic influences of my environment and concentrated on reading scientific material. He continued to appear temperate and modest in his behaviour but soon one of his lady professors appeared to monopolise his emotional life and distracted him substantially from the theory of psychopathology during private tuition. Gradually after our joint voyage into the world of science we began to drift apart; each following his own route. Mitko halted at the threshold of theoretical physics and refused to go any further and I in turn attached little importance to the psychology and psychiatry that were so fascinating to him.

During our scientific meanderings in recent years the issues I discussed with Mitko had gradually extended beyond being a pastime and for me had become the dominant influence. I systematically absorbed books on theoretical physics, theoretical mathematics and informatics. My hobby was to contemplate the challenge of building a new four-stroke internal combustion engine. During the evening as I returned home, bored by the Tyrolese, I would spend hours poring over my books and would finally fall asleep over my drawings of the new engine.

The agony of dawdling through my studies and wasting my time in the process became more unbearable by the day. However it seemed pointless to me to change my course of studies again and to devote myself to physics. Deep within me I was determined that I must defect and planned to do it finally during the next holiday period. At these troubled times the Academy of Fine Arts was indeed the most suitable place for me to be.

My grandmother energetically continued to pursue her life in California. When in Palm Springs she met a Bulgarian who had emigrated to the United States in 1924. Although he was almost eighty and my grandmother about sixty-seven, they announced their intention to marry. She always thought of me and wrote lovingly every week. We had had long discussions about the future before she left Sofia but it seemed at that time quite out of the question for me to travel abroad. Before she left, Grandmother consulted her astrologer in the same way that she had done throughout the last thirty years and in her letters insisted that I should do the same. My grandmother was my financial support at this stage and announced her intention to send money for me to buy a new car. I wrote to her not to make haste and agreed to go and consult Victoria the fortune-teller in whose prophecies my grandmother so staunchly believed.

Victoria's address was in one of the old neighbourhoods of Sofia, a tumbledown collection of prewar housing in poor repair and decoration. On the fourth floor after a long climb a door opened and a very old woman invited me into a tiny drawing room crammed with ancient furniture. She asked me to drink a cup of thick Turkish coffee and to invert the cup so that she could tell my fortune by studying the configuration of the coffee grounds. Victoria, who must have been well into her seventies and appeared to be almost blind, hardly looked at the cup that she held in her hand. I was surprised that she knew immediately who I was and what I had come for. She also knew that I had a spontaneous urge to light a cigarette. There was something mystical in her intuition but her prophecy was definite and assured:

Profession and Hobby

there was no sign of an open road. I would not be able to leave Bulgaria now nor in the years to come.

In fact a further twenty years were to pass before I succeeded in leaving and she said then I would have great success at the steering wheel of a car. My affairs with women would be transitory and it was not until far into the future that a lasting marriage would be made.

Having returned to street level I lit up a cigarette and rejected her prophecy. I refused to accept that my life might be so rigidly defined and promised myself that I would soon defect. However the old fortune-teller Victoria proved to be right.

In the summer the Tyrolese took me to the seaside. We went to Sozopol, a little town of old wooden houses situated on a tiny peninsula on the south coast of the Black Sea. It was a favourite place for actors and artists. The pretty Tyrolese mixed with all sorts of people and I found that rather tiring. There was an Austrian girl there on an exchange visit, there were numerous rather superior and snobbish types and some anonymous but apparently influential big shots known to her mother. The Tyrolese drank heavily and became unbearable. Instead of having a rest I was now so confused that after a week I simply dropped everything and returned to Sofia.

I now knew what I was going to do. Once again I applied for a permit to travel via Yugoslavia and waited for the result. This time however my plan failed. I received a permit allowing me to travel only via Rumania. Were there new rules or was I now under suspicion? Perhaps both possibilities were true. Defection via Yugoslavia had become rather too popular and my file with the State Security would not have become any more confidence-inspiring over recent years.

This situation made me apprehensive and I considered various alternative plans for defection. Unfortunately there were few alternatives available. For people like me there was simply no way of penetrating the Iron Curtain. Throughout the *socialist camp* as the system was known there were many people desperate and ready to do anything for the opportunity to successfully defect. Some resorted to strange inventions; East Germans built balloons secretly at home and tried to fly over the border. A Bulgarian had even succeeded in flying across Yugoslavia with a self-made delta-wing aircraft.

My brother continued to live with his wife's family; minor communist functionaries from an Orthodox background. Lack of privacy in the flat and different attitudes weighed heavily on all. I advanced the idea of continuing my studies abroad, for example by attempting to enter a Yugoslav university. If successful my brother could take over my room in our flat. It seemed to be worth trying and after endless warnings against defection one of his wife's relatives arranged a permit for me to travel to Yugoslavia. Finally the anxiously-awaited piece of paper with signature and seal came into my possession. I realised that this was probably my last opportunity to obtain a permit to travel.

A few days later the Soviet army entered Czechoslovakia to suppress the *Prague Spring*. A contingent of Bulgarian soldiers was sent together with military units from other East European countries. With total disregard for the sensitivities of the world outside the machinery of Leonid Brezhnev's *real socialism* was alerted to sharpen the regimes of all Communist states.

I felt that I was running out of time during those tense weeks. On a nice sunny day at the end of August I bought a ticket, packed a few possessions and prepared myself to take the night train. Late in the afternoon I went out for a last walk. Once downstairs I hesitated for a few seconds to consider the trifling question of which direction to take - should I walk to right or left? In the end I decided to turn left round the corner to a café; *Shapkite* (*The Hats*), where I often sat on the terrace. That apparently insignificant decision in fact changed my life dramatically.

As I turned the corner I spied Rositsa, the unusual girl with freckles and greenish eyes who had failed the entrance examinations of the Academy of Fine Arts. Since then I had only met her once at a party but she had impressed me with her artistic nature and her absurd sense of humour. Again we had felt strongly attracted to each other but she was then still involved with a boyfriend.

This time however she seemed excited to see me and we began to talk. She told me right away that she had wished that she could see me again. Her boyfriend had defected to Italy some weeks ago and she was now alone. A few hours later I confessed to her that I had to catch a train at midnight. She had accompanied me to my little attic and when she heard that, she began to sob. I was twenty-four and my relations with girls so far had only given me a sad and lonely feeling of spiritual incompatibility.

My brief contact with Rositsa and the feelings that I experienced at this time introduced me to a deep sense of intimacy that I had not known before. I attempted to resist the feeling but was overwhelmed by my spontaneous reaction. I was frank with her and told her I had no interest in continuing to live in Bulgaria. The only prospect that I could offer her was to share my defection if she wished to join me and had enough courage for it. Once abroad we would see what might transpire. She immediately accepted my offer and suggested that we should attempt to cross the border together.

This was insane.

I understood that it was extremely difficult to cross the Yugoslavian border illegally and I was aware that there were many uncertainties. In my plans I had even considered studying in Zagreb if that would give me a better chance of escaping to the West. Of course I knew very little of Rositsa and had no understanding of her ability and desire to take part in such a hazardous venture. I was in too much of a hurry to consider things properly and was forced to make a hasty decision. I followed the dictates of my heart.

I immediately postponed my departure and Rositsa applied for a permit to travel to Poland. After two weeks of nerve-racking suspense she received a permit to travel via Yugoslavia which added a moment of exultation to the cocktail of emotions surrounding my relationship with Rositsa. Without further delay we took the night train and together crossed the Bulgarian border on our way to an uncertain future.

This time I had attempted to study more opportunities for defection via Yugoslavia. However the Soviet occupation of Czechoslovakia and the acquisition of my unexpected partner in the venture changed everything. In Belgrade we encountered thousands of Czech citizens - often whole families with children - queueing at the West European embassies in a frantic attempt to obtain a means of leaving the country. The sympathy and moral support offered by Yugoslavians was tempered by fears that any official government support or the granting of an automatic passage to the free world would provoke a Soviet occupation of Yugoslavia, too.

My plan of defection was based on my decision to seek out a
journalist in Zagreb whom I had earlier met in Sofia. I intended to pick up more information from him.

I was unable to find the journalist I knew but chanced upon a colleague who received us warmly. He looked into all the possibilities of asking for political asylum or an exit permit to the West, but in the shadow of the Soviet occupation of Czechoslovakia the only way open to us was to defect by crossing the border illegally. Zagreb was thronged with

Profession and Hobby

Czechs trying to escape and from some of them I learned that it was impossible to cross at Trieste - many had been caught and sent back. Wandering in the streets of Zagreb we exchanged the latest rumours with Czech families we already knew. Some of them planned to cross the frontier at Maribor, a border city on the Austrian frontier. There was little time left to consider the position. I bought tickets to Vienna and Rositsa and I boarded the night train for Maribor.

The train was crowded with Czechs; usually families with small children and grandparents determined to cross the frontier. They were exhausted, loaded with luggage and in a state hovering between despair and hope. I simply could not imagine who could unfeelingly halt them at the border of a country whose citizens were free to travel throughout the world. Perhaps impelled by a desire to share their destiny I suggested to Rositsa that we should stay on the train like everybody else to see whether we would be allowed to cross officially or not. Rositsa and I were the only passengers in a compartment in the last, nearly deserted carriage. The steady rhythm of the train did nothing to ease our tension. We sat silently while I constantly consulted my wristwatch. The compartments next to us were dark so I turned off our lights to judge the result. The darkness did not seem to offer cover but there was space beneath the seats where we could hide, although in discomfort. A passer-by in the corridor would have difficulty in seeing us jammed under the seats. We could throw our luggage out of the window to complete the impression of emptiness.

I offered my plan to Rositsa as a possible means of avoiding a border check but we were unable to reach a decision and just sat waiting to see what would happen. The train halted at the border and the long wait began. Eventually we heard scuffling outside and realized that the border police were ignoring the frantic pleas of the Czechs on board who refused to leave and eventually had to be pulled from the train one by one.

As the approaching police came nearer and ejected some of the passengers from the carriage next to ours, Rositsa, with tears in her eyes suggested that we hide under the seats and switch off the lights. It seemed to us that this was our only chance of success. I sat contemplating the situation but had not moved when the police arrived at our compartment. The exhausted policeman was surprised to find two Bulgarians greeting him, but he was adamant.

Bulgaria had not been invaded or occupied and we did not offer the convincing arguments of the Czechs who had been pulled out of the train. We were there and then forced to get out on to the platform despite Rositsa's tears and as we stood there we realized that we were the last refugees to leave the rapidly departing train. If we had hidden under the seats we would now have been on our way to an Austrian emigration camp. As I watched the lights of our train recede, I felt an agonizing pang of disappointment at having missed my chance. But not for a single moment did I appreciate that it would take me another twenty years before I would pass through the Iron Curtain that I had now so nearly reached. I regarded this incident as yet another failed attempt. On the following day we would make a new start and would have more luck. How wrong I was.

A railway worker advised us to spend a night at the station trying to find a freight train. We passed a sleepless night and in the morning Rositsa was totally exhausted and irritable. I was unable to persuade her to get on a freight car and began to doubt whether she was strong enough to undergo such hardship. Nevertheless later in the day she agreed to walk in an effort to hitch a ride across the border in the hope that the border guards would not check a passing vehicle.

We walked for a few miles between sunny hills, meadows and forests. We met a peasant woman who gave us a discouraging answer to our request for directions. She said the border was somewhere up in the mountains and guarded by dogs and soldiers instructed to shoot escapers on the spot. The only car that stopped in response to our signals contained two Indians who were unable to understand our request for help.

This was the end of our adventure. Rositsa gave up and sank into depression. She refused to continue the attempt to defect and insisted that the only thing she wanted to do was to go home. However I knew that if I returned to Bulgaria I would never again see the border to the West. As we returned to Zagreb I tried to persuade Rositsa that we must once again try to flee on the train to Maribor but she would have nothing of it. This meant that I was now faced with the difficult choice of following my newly-found ideal girlfriend or to undertake a fresh attempt to cross the Yugoslavian border against all odds. After much inner turmoil I surrendered and returned to Sofia with Rositsa.

At the beginning of the new year I was in great trouble. I had missed many of my classes and it took a lot of effort to restore the situation. I gradually came to appreciate the reality of six months ago when instead of carrying out my plan to defect I had ended up with a new girlfriend. Since it was quite impossible for me to emigrate now, I put my worries on one side for the time being and lived through that period in an emotional state of mind. Originally I had seen Rositsa as the girl of my dreams but she had now entered my life as a real human being and although in fact far removed from my ideal I found myself becoming seriously involved with her.

Rositsa was plagued by many small problems and a few more serious ones. They were all founded on her failure to obtain a place at the Academy of Fine Arts and because she was such a difficult person to live with. She had a fine intellect and all the talent and characteristics of a creative artist; liking to shock others with her unrestrained and often outrageous behaviour. She was nervous and highly strung, and would sometimes drink heavily and lose all sense of proportion. But nevertheless she had a fine sense of humour, was charming and original in spirit and appealed to all with her infectious laughter.

We floated in a dreamlike world and the episode in Maribor was a private secret shared in the knowledge that none of our friends would understand it even if they ever suspected that it had happened. Yet it was around this shared experience that dangerous feelings began to surface. On every occasion when I gently raised the subject of a possible future defection Rositsa would become agitated and refuse to discuss it. Sometimes she just got drunk. It became abundantly clear that the subject was taboo and she did not wish to even consider a new attempt to defect. As I could do very little about it at that time I simply avoided mentioning it in order not to provoke unnecessary scenes.

On the other hand, once I had come to terms with things as they were I decided to waste no more time by making use of the encouraging conditions of my studies to concentrate further on the theoretical physics that continued to attract me deeply. My tiny attic gradually became the centre of my life as I spent the majority of my day there reading and re-reading the brilliant *Lectures on Physics* by my now favourite teacher Feynman whose work I had recently discovered. Rositsa would come to my room and often talk me into going out with her but I always rushed back home as I was eager to continue my work. The little attic became progressively crammed with books on quantum mechanics, mathematics and various subjects related to physics. Rositsa complained ironically that she was a fool to think she was in love with an artist.

One day I asked myself what was I actually trying to achieve sitting there alone among all those books on theoretical physics in my tiny attic? Swept along by my intuitive research I had reached the boundaries of the understanding of elementary particles offered by modern physics. Schrödinger and Heisenberg had described the behaviour of such particles in mathematical terms as early as the Twenties and their work was still regarded as the basic theory. One of the problems of that so-called quantum mechanics theory was that the phenomena it described were without a visual model. The theory in fact represents an abstract system of the calculation of probabilities that fails to provide a clear notion of what these particles actually do. This has given rise to prolonged and heated discussion but many scientists consider human imagination incapable of progressing beyond certain clearly defined limits.

At the age of twenty-five I now had an unfavourable file with State Security and was ever more desperate to find an opportunity to flee the country. Hidden in my tiny attic in the centre of Sofia and feeling a deepening claustrophobic abyss between me and the reality outside I became captivated by one of the fundamental theoretical problems of physics and was spending all my energy and attention in its exploration. I asked myself why I did so.

I have no logical answer to that question. Perhaps it was that I just felt it to be the most interesting and pleasant thing to do at the time. I gradually moved further and further into a subject that was entirely abstract and totally removed from the reality of daily life, but on the other hand offering breathtaking beauty and space for the imagination. The normal relationship between logic and experiment did not apply in this case and tempted by the intellectual puzzle I had set myself I began to consider a new theory which might interpret quantum phenomena.

I searched for books and papers on the subject. It was fortunate that a large volume of work on that subject was translated into Russian; everything related to nuclear physics being given the greatest attention and highest priority in view of its military applications. Thousands of students in the Soviet Union and the communist satellite countries were trained in nuclear physics to follow the latest theories published in scientific circles throughout the world. No boundaries or barriers were to be applied to human thought. It is indeed ironical that the greatest ideological dissent and protest against the Communist system emanated from nuclear physicists trained to ensure military supremacy over the West.

During the following years my intellectual activity was concentrated on quantum mechanics and this seemed so worthwhile to me that it prevented the passage of time from seeming wasteful. In the meantime I continued to study at the Academy of Fine Arts and regarded my work on car design as a pleasant relaxation made possible by the freedom and spare time allowed by my life as a student.

My personal relationship with Rositsa progressively foundered on the problems that we had encountered from the outset. She made two unsuccessful attempts to obtain a place at the Academy while completing a course in photography. When I brought up the subject of future emigration she would immediately dismiss it and fly into a rage regardless of whether she was sober or not.

My grandmother announced her marriage to Alexander Nikolov, a Bulgarian-American, in Palm Springs, California. She returned home for a holiday and took stock of our situation which had changed considerably since her departure. She voiced her disapproval of my brother's marriage and did not take to Rositsa. Her intention to buy me a new car was now realized with the gift of a Renault 8 which brought a new excitement tempered by the realisation that I would not be able to use it abroad as an emigré.

Strange changes affected my friend Mitko. He ceased reading scientific books although he listened carefully to me when I described my latest investigations in the field of quantum mechanics. I frequently noticed his own confused meandering in completely different areas. He was now deeply in love with his lady professor of psychopathology and in a strange voice would share with me elements of his relationship with her that seemed quite absurd. After taking part in voluntary experiments with drugs he became progressively psychotic. I felt deeply troubled by the destruction of his fine mind but unable to help him in his tormented state.

At that time Bobby continued his studies in Moscow and we only met during his brief holidays. I maintained contact with another of my former classmates, Branimir, who although married continued to work and follow a part-time course in engineering studies. He was the only one of my circle with whom I continued to share my intellectual scientific journeys and my desire to invent a new four-stroke engine.

In the meantime Grandmother and her new husband returned to Sofia and they purchased a flat in the newly developed prefabricated blocks in *Mladost*, the housing estate near my former educational institute. I moved in with them and they bought me a new car, an amazingly beautiful red Renault 16TS. For most Bulgarians such a car was an unattainable dream. Sadly, a few months after his return, my grandmother's new husband who had been away from Sofia for half a century, died.

During my last year at the Academy I once again raised with myself the matter of emigration. I had delayed it until after my graduation because I had not yet seen a single suitable opportunity. My mind was concentrated in the summer of 1971 when Rositsa announced that she was pregnant. I had never considered that I might marry and settle down with a wife and child before emigrating. The future ahead saddened me and I felt confronted by numerous problems that I had never considered before. I could not see how any of them could be solved and this made me feel extremely confused. I desperately sought a new plan for my future life. I then decided to develop the concept of one of the four-stroke engines that had always occupied my mind although an inner voice told me that I should wait before trying to harvest the as yet unripened fruit of my talent as an inventor.

I developed an idea inspired by the Wankel rotary engine and succeeded in persuading Branimir to share my enthusiasm for it. We jointly filed for a certificate of copyright and began to work on the project.

To be a professional inventor in Eastern Europe offered very little chance of success and would certainly hardly provide a living. Lenin had already ensured that under the Communist yoke the expropriation of capital and the means of production by the state ensured that inventions were the property of the State, too. As a result, the intellectual *kolkhoz* of inventors was as ineffective as any other collective and certainly a great deal madder. The Institute for Inventions was not so much a patent agency as an organisation intended to apply useful inventions within state companies that were not in the slightest bit interested in them. No-one could possibly make a living from the fruits of invention. In cases where there was a little success the designer might receive a few inconsequential privileges, decorations and modest financial rewards hardly enough to buy a car and then only if his invention had resulted in profits of millions to the State. Understandably there were only one or two cases of success in this field whilst the win-

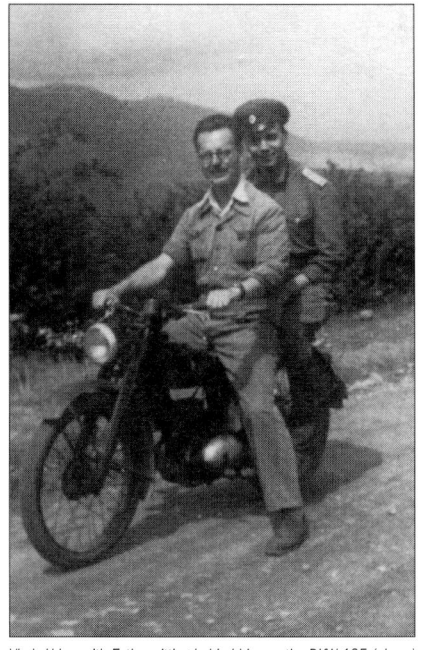

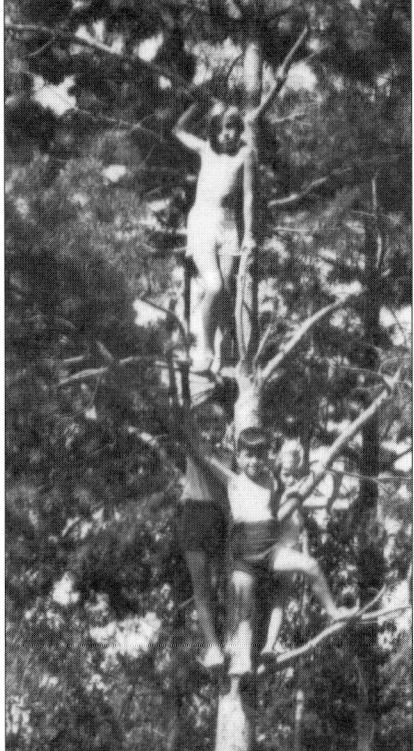

Vlady Udrev with Father sitting behind him on the DKW 125 (above)

Adriana high up a tree with me, my brother and Rosalina below her, in a Boyana meadow (right)

Shortly before my arrest in 1961, showing an automobile catalogue to Bobby (22) (below)

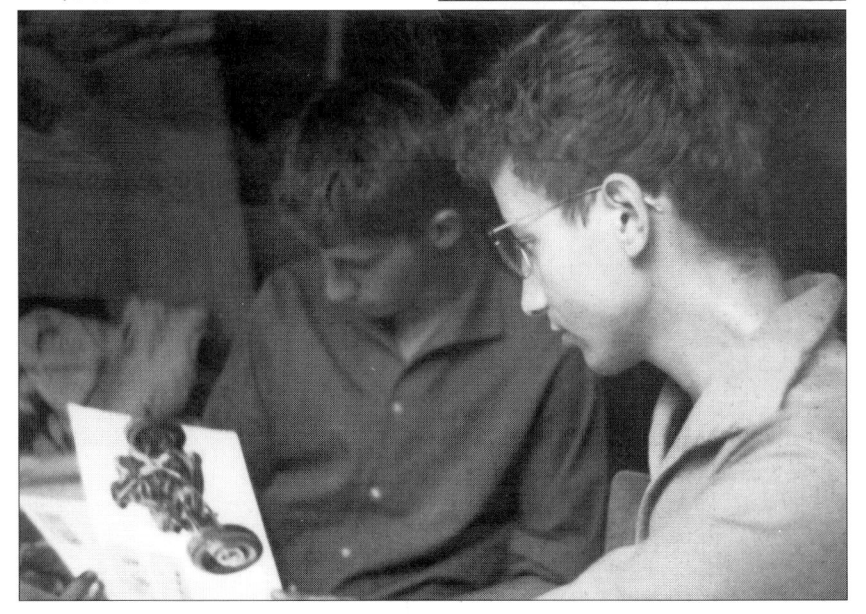

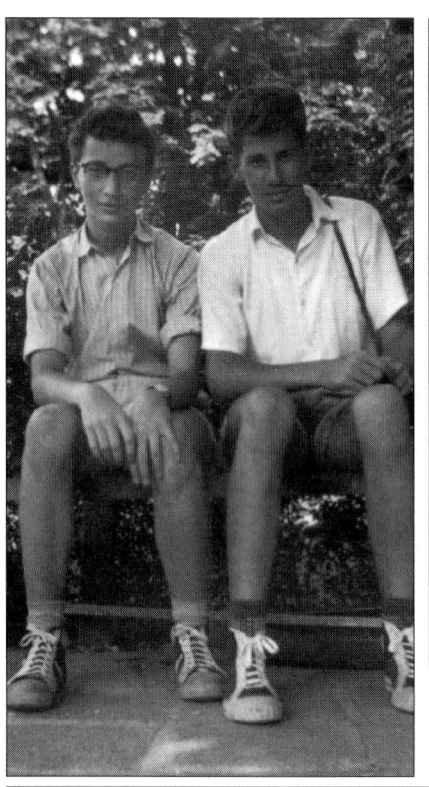

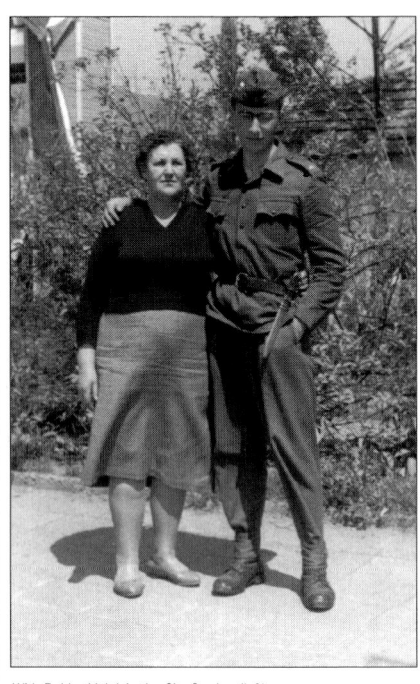

With Bobby (right) in the City Garden (left)

Grandmother visited me at the garrison before leaving for California (above)

Army days - I am third from left (below)

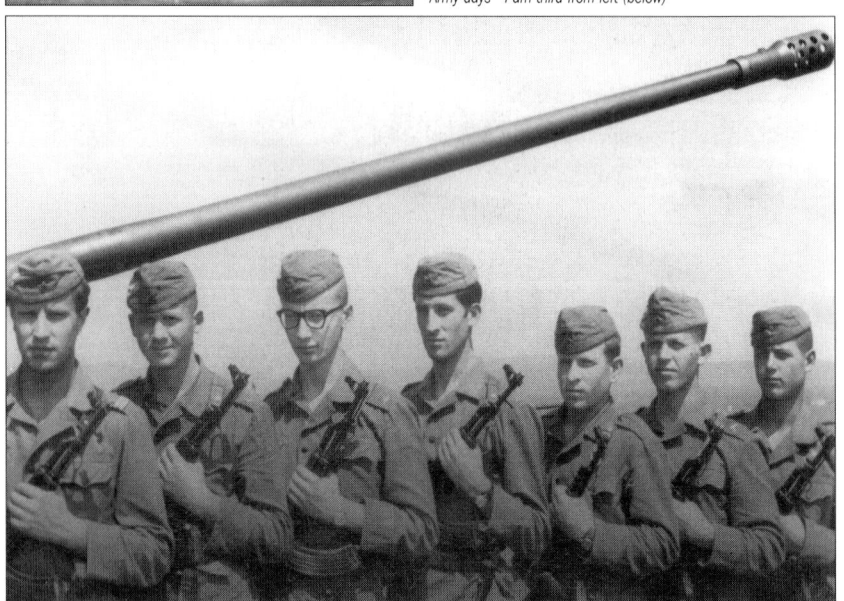

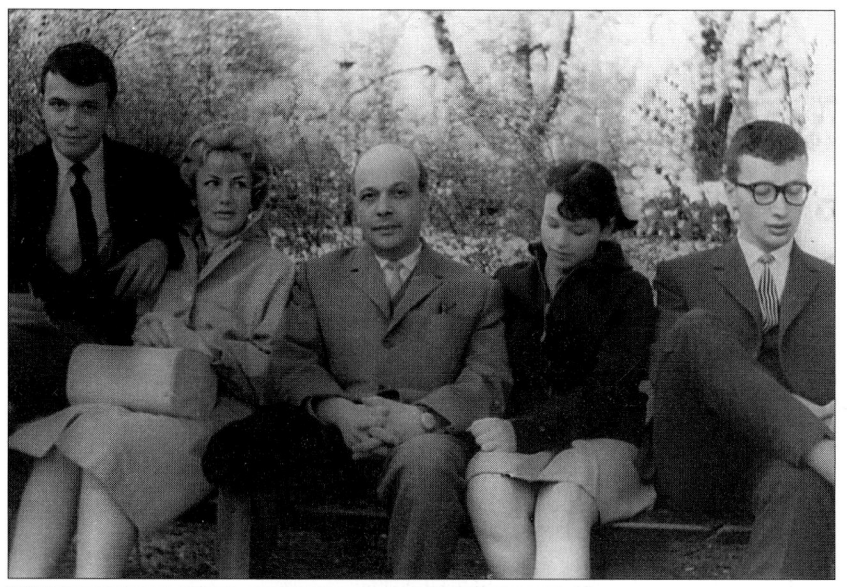

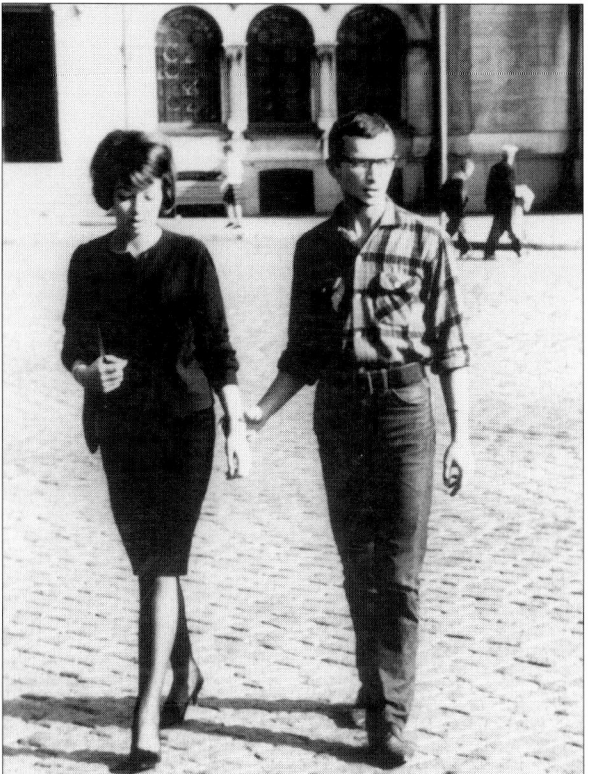

*The Family Antonov in 1964:
(Left to right) my brother, parents,
sister and I*

*Vera and I passing the Alexander
Nevski cathedral*

Student days with the white Renault 8

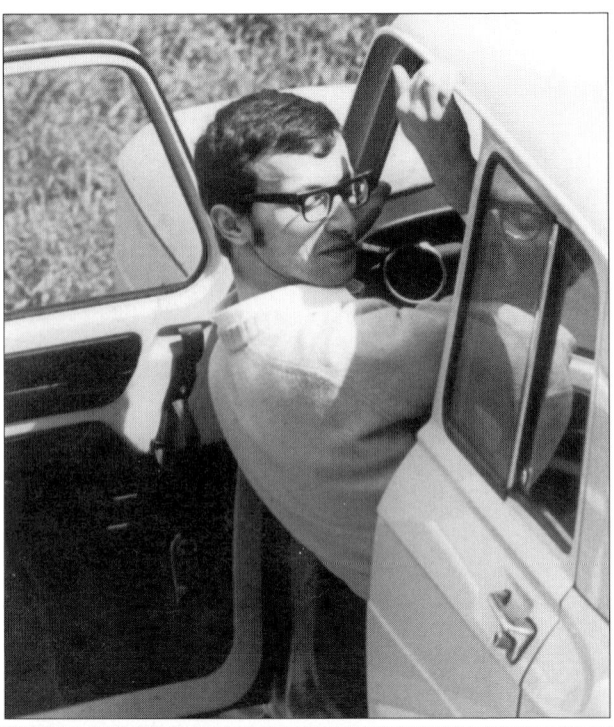

Rositsa

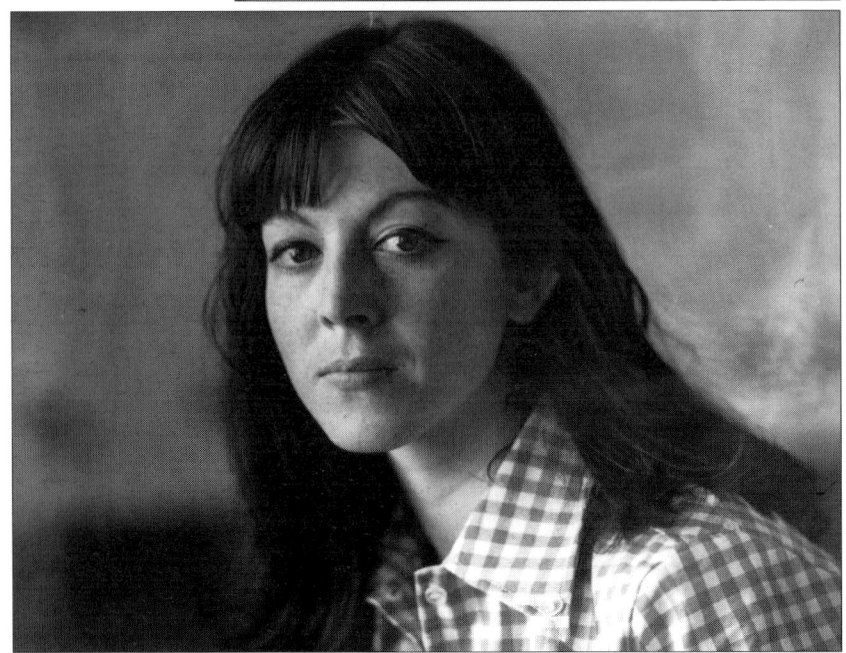

Profession and Hobby

ning prize in the state lottery seemed to increase all the time. Deprived of the opportunity of testing their inventions in a practical application, many thousands of fanatical inventors were locked in a desperate war of correspondence with the Institute for Inventions.

Judged against that background, my initiative had no basis in logic. Moreover the search for a new engine seemed in the same class as the quest for perpetual motion. Bulgaria did not even have a car industry. Nevertheless all inventors are out of touch with reality - on occasions at least - and I was certainly no exception to the rule.

Despite the apparent lack of a local market for it, the parts for my engine were manufactured in a plant in Varna and assembled according to my design. Unfortunately the result failed to function as a prime mover and was more of a pump spraying a cloud of petrol and oil all over the workshop. This resulted in a swift temporary conclusion of testing until the autumn when after my wedding I was able to resume work on the engine at Varna and to take the opportunity to enjoy a few months of pleasant walks along the Black Sea coast.

On 5th February 1972 my son Viktor was born.

Despite the great confusion surrounding me I was still absorbed in the world of theoretical physics where I felt that I had made some very important discoveries hinting at a new theory in the world of physics: three centuries ago Isaac Newton had created the first modern scientific theory determining the changing position of an object in relation to change in time. Newton regarded the two notions - space and time - as *absolute*. In that sense space resembles a rectangular room with the walls, ceiling and floor reaching far into infinity. The entire world and all existing objects are situated within and their form and position is determined by their three projections on the surfaces of the room.

As far as time is concerned, it passes through that infinitely large room and may be measured at any point at a given moment. This seems so self-evident as to be tautological. But from a different perspective it becomes possible to understand that science does not examine anything not situated in the infinitely large room and within the time passing in that room. So far science has paid little attention to events taking place outside the infinitely large room. Those obvious views about the infinitely large room and the time elapsing within it have been profoundly changed by the work of Einstein. Because of the limited speed of light, the speed and chronology of time become relative concepts while the infinitely large room no longer appears to be rectilinear and rectangular.

In the study of elementary particles, quantum mechanics makes use of Newton's view of the infinitely large room and more precisely a system of mathematics based on that view, assuming that space and time may be divided into infinitely small units.

One day I came to consider a different way of describing what happens to elementary particles. If they could be described without the notion of space and time, then space and time could be perceived as consequences of what happened to elementary particles. My idea was basically quite simple. However the phenomena and experiments in the world of quanta are so far removed from ordinary thought that it is impossible to describe such ideas without first entering various scientific fields and even the basics of mathematics.

Contemplation of my new idea brought me the greatest possible satisfaction and I continued further in various scientific fields in order to explore it as thoroughly as possible. It became obvious too that I was now quite far removed from what was going on around me in the world because of my intellectual activities. I had travelled a long way alone in order to develop a new scientific concept and it was therefore time to ask myself what I should do in the future. My failure so far to emigrate and the circumstances in which I lived kept me yet further away from my dream of studying at a university in California. What should I do?

I attended a seminar on theoretical physics attended by the few intellectuals working in that field. Among them was the Bulgarian doyen of physics, Christo Christov, a selection of professors and lecturers from the University of Sofia and a group of other physicists interested in or already working on the theory of physics. This seminar was presided over by Professor Azarya Polikarov. I found myself to be the youngest in the assembly.

The participants presented papers that later would be published in the first collection of articles on theoretical physics in Bulgaria. Most of these papers were concerned with quantum mechanics. Under the influence of Soviet science some authors examined the philosophical problems created by Marxist dogma, but all participants held the most advanced views on modern physics and were entirely dedicated to their work. The seminar began in 1971 and continued for more than a year with each paper followed by heated discussion.

I was now so dedicated to working on my new theory that I could not avoid taking part in the discussions following the presentation of each paper. On one day after a heated exchange between one of the participants and me, Professor Polikarov observed that it was easy to criticize a thesis but more difficult to launch and defend one. I therefore took up the gauntlet, and offered to present a paper in order to provide my audience with the opportunity to examine it critically. My offer was accepted immediately.

Without delay I set about writing my paper in order to present my theories as clearly as possible although this was all happening at the time my son Viktor was born. All participants in the seminar received a copy of my paper before the meeting where I read my work calmly only to immediately find myself at the centre of a furious discussion.

My idea was a radical one concerning the very basis of the theory of quantum mechanics. The immediate reaction from my audience was to point out inconsistencies between my theories and existing publications on the subject but I managed to pass that test with flying colours and the discussion soon became calmer. I then suddenly received the enthusiastic support and recognition of Professor Strigachev, head of the department of nuclear physics at the University of Sofia who had just come home after spending two years at Princeton University. He accepted my theory and took my side. A second meeting dedicated only to the discussion of my paper ended with full recognition being accorded to me in a spirit of scientific triumph. Although my idea was still subject to argument my paper would be published in the first Bulgarian miscellany of articles on theoretical physics.

Immediately after the meeting Professor Strigachev invited me to his department. We had a long discussion of our views on the theory of physics and at the end I received an offer which presented me with a difficult choice. The Professor invited me to work as his assistant at the department of nuclear physics.

Having left the faculty of physics where my sister - now influenced by me - was studying nuclear physics, I relaxed in the dark red Renault 16 and pondered the situation for some time before starting the engine. Einstein had published his first article at the age of twenty-seven and defected from Nazi Germany at the age of forty-two. I was twenty-eight but not content to wait that long.

Chapter Six
Wandering in a Maze

I now adopted a new emigration strategy. In an attempt to be practical I abandoned the idea of making a living from theoretical physics, engineering invention or motorcar design. I decided to enter the film industry as an art director.

Shortly before the publication of my paper on theoretical physics, Yakim Yakimov, a film director, offered me the opportunity to work on a three-part TV series. *The Blue Lamp* was about a group of courageous policemen maintaining public order. Yakim gave me the screenplays and told me that he would wait for my answer.

While reading these texts I was overcome by a strong desire to hurl them into the trash can. Two of the screenplays were written by the dictator Zhivkov's son-in-law Slavkov. Slavkov was a notorious playboy and highly experienced in commercial fraud. He made good use of his wife's influential family and had established his career as the head of national television. Now he had the impertinence to stitch together a couple of miserable texts in pursuit of money and fame. One of his appalling scenarios for *The Blue Lamp* related the story of a corrupt Bulgarian scientist spying for the West. Under instruction from his bosses the scientist is on the point of carrying out a subversive act involving setting fire to his institute which has recently discovered a cancer drug whose secret he has already betrayed. One night the evil scientist pours petrol over the floor of the institute. Above him probably on the roof of the building there is a huge oil tank supplying the central heating system. At this very moment a courageous policeman fortuitously passes by on his way to a birthday party. As he walks along the quiet street he notices a suspicious movement; an ape has escaped from a cage of animals used for scientific experiment and is running amok in the corridors. A dead man is slumped in the porter's office at the entrance to the building. Without hesitation the policeman leaps into the lake of fuel oil, is attacked by the treacherous scientist but in some miraculous way the policeman succeeds in turning off an incandescent heating element a few inches above the rising fuel oil.

The only item in this plot that interested me was the scene where the scientist was recruited for espionage by a couple of suspicious-looking characters. In the script the scene was described as a bustling Western city and this meant that the crew could justify shooting the scenes in Vienna. If I worked on the film I would be among the first to go. This caused me to deliberate for some time as I turned over the pages of the script. The scene with the scientist and his Viennese treachery was in the third episode. Before shooting that we had to complete the first episode in which the same courageous, shrewd policeman arrested an international female terrorist by identifying a blue parrot tattooed on her bosom. I knew all too well that I would only be given the opportunity to travel to Vienna after having worked for at least a year on tattooed parrots, experimental apes and other products of the Socialist film industry. This therefore appeared to be my only realistic chance of defection and in the end I signed a contract with the studios of Feature Films situated in Boyana, the town that had fascinated me in my childhood.

It was indeed a great privilege to work at The Film Centre as the studios were called. In common with all other artistic endeavour, the cinema was generously subsidised by the State and was not required to operate profitably. Film industry people passed their time in long relaxing holidays at the best hotels in the country, enjoyed their fill of good food and wine and never ceased complaining of being misunderstood and generally badly treated. Film directors were the most privileged members of this group; some of them became spoilt, despotic frauds. They were all of course Party members with an impeccable background, an unimpeachable record of Party activities and the correct political views; they were members of the *nomenclatura*, those who enjoyed the complete confidence of the communist authorities.

Yakim Yakimov was a short, smiling man with modest manners and the subtle charisma of pensive but hesitant people. It was difficult to take him seriously as he was totally different from his fellow film directors. Having made a few films ten years earlier he had produced nothing since and had in fact wasted the intervening years in long fruitless discussions of totally worthless screenplays. Now he was forced to face the choice of either accepting the appalling screenplay of *The Blue Lamp* or finally to withdraw into oblivion, pushed by his fellow directors. Yakim was also tempted by the possibility of earning some money from the film to supplement the salary of his idle years.

Yakim liked and respected me and took my comments on the screenplays seriously even though they sometimes threatened to persuade him to abandon the whole project. But then, thinking of his wife and the fuss that she would make if he continued in his idle ways he quickly changed his mind. His wife Chonka was a young, energetic and sturdy peasant girl who had made a career as a singer of Bulgarian folk songs. She had little patience with her husband and his indecisive behaviour.

I had to be careful. Sometimes it was difficult for me to conceal my true motives for taking part in that mad circus. I kept reminding myself that it would be worthwhile to put up a convincing act as a hard-working art director because the film consultants from the police and Chonka's friends were influential enough to help me on that dream trip to Vienna. Besides my part in the film-making was so easy and inconsequential that I sometimes felt rather ashamed about it.

I would turn up at the studios in the morning to join in pointless discussions over vast quantities of coffee. During the early afternoon everybody would leave and Yakim went home to consider the screenplays. We spent a few weeks at a hotel in the Vitosha mountains near Sofia working on the shooting script and travelled across country searching vainly for suitable locations for the filming. At the same miserably slow pace Yakim constantly brooded over his choice of actors and even over the extras who would appear only for a few seconds in some idiotic scene.

There was little for me to do at that stage of the absurd preparations. Nevertheless Yakim sought my opinion over every pointless detail and I did my very best to appear committed. My salary hardly improved my standard of living and after our son was born, Rositsa and I moved into my grandmother's flat.

Now well into her seventies, my grandmother was as vigorous and stubborn as ever. She had achieved what would seem impossible for most people at that time. She received a pension of a few hundred dollars from the US that amounted to approximately ten times my own salary. To buy a flat like hers with Bulgarian currency would mean waiting dozens of years.   After buying the impressive Renault 16 for me, Grandmother gave the old Renault 8 to my brother. Still both cars were nominally in her possession and she liked to remind us all of the fact.

My grandmother was not an easy person to live with. She had provided me with a home and all that she expected in return was to see me achieve success in life. In her eyes I remained the young naive rather helpless boy whom she loved so much. My relationship with her which had been difficult since my childhood now worsened when I brought my family to live in her flat.

It only required a few weeks for Grandmother and Rositsa to reach a state of hostility. My efforts to mediate and resolve the problems failed and soon their heated arguments caused irreparable damage. Eventually Rositsa took Viktor with her and returned to her parents who lived in a small overcrowded house lacking all the facilities to bring up a baby.

Behind the impressive facade of my Grandmother's wealth I still lacked confidence. I was convinced that Rositsa's departure from the flat was only the beginning and that other disasters would soon follow.

The frontier at Maribor that Rositsa and I had failed to cross in the autumn of 1968 now came between us. Despite my innumerable efforts to persuade Rositsa to change her mind and agree to leave the country she became progressively more intolerant and irritable whenever I so much as hinted at a new attempt to defect. The gap between us had steadily widened and in fact we were no longer close by the time that she became pregnant and we were forced to marry. Viktor's birth did not alter Rositsa's Bohemian lifestyle. I did my best to help her and to prepare her for future emigration although it seemed a hopeless task. In the end I had to admit that even I had abandoned hope that she might change her mind.

In those days I spent a good deal of time with Bobby discussing a range of subjects like old times. Soon after the birth of his daughter, Bobby discovered that he could no longer live with his wife and left her. After graduating in Moscow he came home to begin divorce proceedings and got involved with another girl. Finally he returned to his wife and a few years later they had a son. He worked at an institute for oil and gas research and lived with his wife and two children in a tiny one-room flat on a housing estate far removed from the city centre. Still Bobby was not a complainer and he enjoyed his job.

I could share my problems with Bobby but did not tell him about my intention to leave the country. We discussed my ideas on quantum physics and my ludicrous film work. We often discussed life in general; Bobby believed that something exciting would soon happen to him, expecting that his life would change dramatically because of a new love affair or better career prospects. But while waiting for this change he never even considered that he could quite simply divorce or emigrate.

Bobby's patience and endurance and his general attitude to life reminded me of how far I had drifted away from what was commonly accepted as a normal life in Bulgaria at the time. He was satisfied with his job and did not appear to covet a house or car, those two essential items for which most Bulgarians had to save and wait for years. When I compared my situation with his I felt alienated. All intellectual activity of the officially censored type allowed seemed to me flimsy and even ridiculous; I sneered at the culture, its docile creators and the authorities who supported it. It was difficult for me to even put up an act as a diligent art director. I was not interested in the flat that my grandmother had decided to leave to me nor in her car. I would happily exchange both together with all my material possessions for a single opportunity to quit Bulgaria. When I thought of my baby son and his bleak future if I failed to emigrate and take him with me I felt sad indeed.

During the 1970s news from the outside world barely trickled into Bulgaria, distorted beyond recognition. The US landing on the moon was dismissed in a couple of lines of small print on the back page of the newspapers with any emphasis laid on the technical problems experienced. All news from the West was relayed in terms of general decay and decline. Eastern European life was inevitably highly praised and the newspapers were packed with reports of the enormous successes with barely any reference to problems, natural disasters and even accidents. Yet most people were directly aware of the wide gap in living standards and technological development between East and West although their understanding of the latter was generally vague and inaccurate. The brighter minds among my peers regarded Western civilization with a childlike fascination that was only stimulated by the censorship and blatant demagogy around us. A feeling of affinity with the West was often manifested in a yearning for material items, since we all felt painfully aware of the material and spiritual poverty of life in the communist world.

I refused to accept the restraints that the communist system would have imposed on me. My thoughts and desires ranged far beyond the spiritual boundaries of communism and I imagined myself competing with the finest minds in the world of ideas. I avidly read all available sources of information in the fields that interested me and frequented those few libraries stocking the very few books and Western magazines that arrived with despairing infrequency. I could spend hours turning the pages of a recent copy of *Quattroruote* and *L'Automobile,* fascinated by the pictures and drawings from another world where even the colours and shapes were so different from the primitive and ugly reality of my surroundings.

Was my concept of the world to which I so eagerly wished to emigrate, realistic? At that time I truly believed that the West offered the only civilization created by free people and I had now chosen to join it. Every time I worked on my theory of physics or on my engine design I felt this conviction more strongly. At times I imagined that I would write a letter to Feynman and send him my new paper on quantum mechanics. I worked late at night on my article and on elaborating my engine design or sketching out car bodies inspired by the great classic motor cars of the 1930s. At that time my personal life became even more ridiculous. The continuing conflict between my wife and my grandmother had reached a point at which there was very little that I could do about it and it created difficulties in my relationship with both. I did my best to make my son Viktor's life more comfortable; taking him in my car to my grandmother's flat for his daily bath. Fortunately it was Rositsa's father Alexander, a quiet man with a kind heart, who took care of him.

In the final scenes of the first episode of the film the international female terrorist was arrested at a lake near Sofia. Besides having to draw a tattooed parrot with a felt-tip pen on her huge bosom, I had a minor role as her stand-in wearing a blonde wig and driving a car because the actress herself had no driving licence. Then the tediously extended period of editing and dubbing the film began and continued throughout the winter.

Finally we began to shoot the film with the betrayal scenes in Vienna. The crew travelled around the country seeking a suitable interior for the scenes of the institute when flooded with fuel oil. The laboratory of a factory in Vidin manufacturing tyres was chosen. I designed the set that would give the laboratory the glamour of an institute capable of developing an important cancer drug but in fact it was nothing more than a few fake sliding doors with secret codes and canvas walls painted with white emulsion.

Wandering in a Maze

I worried whether I could develop the image of a hard-working art director sufficiently trustworthy to be allowed to travel to Vienna despite the existence of a far from satisfactory file in the police archives. Yakim had no influence within the system to obtain a permit for me and I had no access to any people of influence who could do it for me. Besides I had a vague premonition that Slavkov, the dictator's son-in-law, might have heard from his numerous informers about my less than flattering views on his screenplays. It was unlikely that he would like me and so I was obliged to wait to see what the future held.

The new cameraman Petko Petkov made no secret of the fact that he had been sent by his friend Slavkov to keep an eye on what was going on on the set and to inform him accordingly. Equally he made no attempt to conceal his particular interest in me and we shared a hotel room during our stay in Vidin. Petko was a large florid man with well-polished manners and a taste for the good life in the film industry. Although we pretended that we were close friends we both knew better. He was a romantic and it became quickly obvious that he was attracted to the script girl Galya, the daughter of one of Bulgaria's famous film producers Borislav Sharaliev, who happened to be the Communist Party secretary at the Film Centre.

I was twenty-nine. In the past few years various girls had been obviously attracted to me and it had become difficult for me to resist female temptation. I had always thought that my guardian angel was strong enough to keep me out of trouble but I was sadly mistaken. For a long time I resisted the advances of girls associated with my friends but at times when left alone with some of them I gave in. Temptation sometimes took me by surprise. On a sunny day I visited someone working at an institute for water supply projects in one of those dull buildings far from the city centre with large windows and scores of employees killing time by idling and drinking coffee. I entered a room and discovered a pretty young brunette in a white overall who seemed so disturbed by my question as to where I could find her colleague that she was at a loss to answer. After a very confused and puzzling discussion words no longer seemed to matter and she left with me. It was all very exciting and she nearly fainted in the car while I kept asking myself what on earth was going on. We met again a couple of times but it was an insane affair in which neither of us could manage to say much.

One sunny day as I drove dangerously fast along the narrow potholed roads on my way to the film set in Vidin I had a distinct feeling that my guardian angel was far from my side. I kept thinking about the pretty secretary at the plant in Vidin who had seemed at a loss when I entered her office. I kept telling myself that I should not think about love affairs as I travelled on my way to Vidin with the intention of presenting myself as a conscientious art director who could be trusted on a trip to Vienna.

Unfortunately my premonition came true. The secretary again did her best to attract me. In fact I was able to resist her albeit with some difficulty, but I succumbed to the advances of a young actress in the local theatre; a girl with cold blue eyes and a dreamy face who wanted to study at the Sofia Film Academy. She coaxed me into staying with her and I was quite embarrassed on the following morning when my roommate the cameraman Petko Petkov did not even trouble to ask me where I had spent the night.

Galya, the scriptgirl Petko was in love with always gave me a wide friendly smile but I made no attempt to seduce her. She was a well-mannered twenty year-old and looked quite attractive in her expensive fashionable dresses but I suspected that she was a communist virgin with a fearsome party secretary of a father who was watching her carefully and who would repel all admirers. I amused myself with flirting with her with a theatrical openness, certain that I had no need of my guardian angel - I felt entirely safe with her since I assumed that she was too prudish and innocent to get such ideas into her pretty head.

We continued to flirt in the same careless way and danced every evening in the restaurant where she appeared with her long dark hair spreading over her shoulders, dressed just like a model girl in a fashion magazine. As we danced to the tune of *Spanish Eyes* I gazed into hers and what I saw there had little to do with communist prudishness. Galya dismissed my affair with the young actress as a frivolity and I told her that people in my situation could expect very little from life. Galya disagreed so I asked her if she would like to invite me to her room for the night.

She did so.

When I knocked at her door I imagined that I was engaged in an innocent joke and did not expect to have any problem in keeping a cool head. How wrong I was; in the morning I awoke in her bed with Galya held tightly in my arms. We probably both realized simultaneously that what had taken place between us might have grave consequences.

I was not mistaken. The days in Vidin were a lovely but fleeting episode in our affair. The town was charming with narrow streets and the relics of what once had been the towers of an old fortress. In the centre of the town I found the house that had once belonged to my grandfather and where my father was born; today it accommodated the theatre club. But all this came to an abrupt end when a few days later we returned to Sofia.

Although I had been included in the list of film crew intended for Vienna by the Feature Film studio, the police passport department refused to issue me with a travel permit. Thus I was scratched from the list. Yakim's wife Chonka went to visit anonymous influential friends but was unable to help me. I never fully excluded the possibility of failure but still the refusal came as a severe shock. People were normally allowed to go abroad on a genuine business trip and similar applications for passports were rarely turned down. This meant that State Security had categorized me as untrustworthy and a potential defector after having routinely investigated my record. The denial of a permit meant that I had lost all chances of ever travelling abroad for any reason.

There was no point in attempting to discover the reason for my failure in that mad world. Perhaps it was connected with my love affairs or my overheard comments on the writings and personality of the President's son-in-law, Slavkov. In any case a file like mine gave me little chance of acceptance by the all-pervasive but invisible state security service. What really counted was my failure to present a convincing performance of a citizen who had fully accepted life under the Communist system. Whenever I occasionally forced myself to play that role, I was miserable.

I immediately resigned from the feature film studio after the refusal of a permit to travel to Vienna. I decided that I would now apply directly to the passport department of the police for a permit although common sense told me that this was a desperate move with no chance of success. However there seemed to be nothing else that I could do and driven into an impossible situation, I had unrealistically imagined that I might possibly succeed. By substituting fantasy for reality I had persuaded myself that I might be allowed to travel abroad for what I called a *private project*; the reason included on my application form.

In 1973 even the simple act of applying for a passport giving the holder the right to travel abroad was an extremely tiresome enterprise. To begin with, the regulation forms of application were not available in the shops supposed to sell them. I was told that they

Wandering in a Maze

had simply run out of stock. Beside this the applicant was obliged to present a dozen other documents issued and verified by various authorities including his present employer. The applicant also needed the guarantee of a foreign citizen that he would be provided with accommodation and money during his stay abroad. A large sign at the passport department announced that only application forms for a visit to a close relative abroad would be accepted. The final act was the announcement by a sullen anonymous female that the applicant had been denied a permit.

I had devised a plan of action intended to get me through that bureaucratic mill. Immediately after tendering my resignation I visited the director of the Centre for Industrial Aesthetics where a few years earlier I had successfully won a competition with my motorcycle design. I offered to work for the Centre in exchange for its support of a private project abroad if I undertook to provide the finance myself. All I needed was an official letter stating that my project was of the greatest significance to Bulgaria's only design centre. The director, a tiny dark man, was a sly and skilful bureaucrat who showed respect for me and in the end accepted my offer. A week later, I had been appointed designer at the Centre of Industrial Aesthetics and held in my hand a letter stating that the Centre had given its consent to my plan for study abroad. I had already attended to the rest of the documents required. A Swedish family I had met at the seaside a year earlier agreed to send me an invitation. Moreover I had my grandmother's financial support in the form of hard currency. Now I had all the necessary papers and finally succeeded in convincing the anonymous employee at the passport department to accept my unusual form of application.

This was the time of the East/West Helsinki conference and Brezhnev's party committee was eager to have the Communist system recognized as a legitimate form of government. The Western countries raised the subject of human rights including the right to travel abroad. This conference had given hope to many people and I was among those who desperately believed in the declarations issued by the West. Should my application be turned down I was determined to write to the appeal committee or to insist on a meeting with the deputy minister as I was told had been successfully done by some. My reasons for wanting to go to the West were reasonable, I thought, and entirely legitimate; although perhaps naive, they still seemed to me sufficiently valid to convince the police functionaries who would soon confront me.

Some time passed before I heard anything from the passport department. While waiting I designed a welding unit and a home heater. Eventually the summons to report to the passport department arrived. At the desk a female employee asked for the letter, put it away and told me that I had been refused permission to travel abroad. No reason was given. I immediately made an appointment with the appeal committee.

While waiting in the room for my turn to appear before the appeal committee I noticed that the majority of the men and women present, who were mostly elderly folk anxious to visit their children abroad, had a short interview and came out weeping. It transpired that the committee was represented by a single bald and overweight man. He confirmed that I had been denied permission to travel abroad and when I tried to explain myself he stood up, opened the door and showed me the way out.

I then made an appointment with the Deputy Minister of the Interior, Zdravko Georgiev. On entering his office I was immediately struck by his enormous ears which projected from both sides of a small, wrinkled face. I had never seen a face like that before. As I presented my case he continually searched for a file on his desk; finally having obviously found the file he opened it, scrutinized a paper and bluntly turned down my request without even offering me the chance to finish what I had intended to say.

It was now the end of the year and also the end of all my hopes. I resigned from the Centre of Industrial Aesthetics having worked there for less than four months. In order to earn some money I accepted a commission to design cars for a merry-go-round. I had fun modelling them after prewar car designs but I still felt deeply unhappy. I could not imagine what I would do. Everything in my life was ephemeral and getting more so all the time.

I now began automatically to think more about the four-stroke engine that had kept my mind busy in a spontaneous inner process that had continued for fifteen years. My imagination constantly examined a series of designs that would offer a variable volume between moving elements. I pursued a solution that could improve the existing four-stroke piston engine and a stubborn inner voice constantly reminded me that one day I would come up with the right idea. It was not only a great pleasure to me to allow my imagination to consider a range of metal parts; I firmly believed that aided by imagination and reflection, the only instruments at my disposal, I could win my lonely struggle with the world's most advanced technologies. This was somewhat over-confident considering the ever-widening gap between reality and my mental processes.

At the beginning of the new year Rositsa began divorce proceedings. My affair with Galya had deeply upset her. A few months later she was granted a divorce and the custody of our two year-old son Viktor. The harmony in our relationship that I had tried to maintain during the previous year was now completely destroyed and Rositsa became unpredictable, unbalanced and hostile to me.

After she moved out I lived in an empty room with nothing but a mattress on the floor. I had no desire for comfort, hated everything including the flat, the housing estate, and even my life there and I argued with my grandmother despite her enormous and continuing support. I tried to explain to her that as I intended to leave the country as soon as possible it was pointless to furnish my room but that only made her more unhappy. She was often angry and lost her temper but then would forgive me and try to bribe me with something she thought that I might like.

My relations with Galya became difficult and I was frequently on the point of ending my relationship with her. However Galya refused to allow this and seemed very much involved with me. Although she understood my problems and supported me in my views which were generally the opposite to hers - such as my determination to defect - I still felt a great gap between us in our attitude to life. She was devoted to her father and her respect for him could not be influenced by her feelings for me.

One of Galya's colleagues introduced me to her husband, Bogomil Terziev. He was an energetic man of about fifty who had once been a cadet at the Military School like my father. His flamboyant personality was at odds with the drab reality of life.

He was an expert in the repair and tuning of violins and had practised the rare trade of *luthier* in Sofia for some time before moving to Zagreb and later to Vienna. He chatted freely, was somewhat vain, quick-tempered and emotional but very easy to get on with. He said right away that he liked me and sympathized with me because of my unsuccessful attempts to defect. He was absolutely convinced that I must go to the West and achieve those things that were beyond me in Bulgaria.

After our first meeting I saw him a couple of times and we had a long discussion. Bogomil offered to help me to leave Bulgaria although I had little illusion about my chances of success. Nevertheless a complicated system of bribery and corruption flourished in the country and many articles that could not be bought could perhaps be obtained in exchange for a favour if one had the right connections. This corrupt network was mainly based on human relationships through relatives and friends and ensured that one could get almost anything which otherwise would be beyond reach. All kinds of things that were never available in Bulgarian shops as well as entry to a university course or even a permit to travel abroad.

The bureaucrats of the State Security formed the peak of that very hierarchical network and Bogomil made no secret of the fact that he had contacts in the right places. However I asked myself whether his contacts would be sufficient and what it was that he was to offer them in return for their favours. But I was hardly in a position to ask questions because I needed Bogomil's help so very much. He assured me that he knew the head of the service issuing travelling permits to East European countries including Yugoslavia. Bogomil went to see him and then told me that he could arrange for a permit by personally guaranteeing me.

Everything now seemed like a dream. I applied for a permit to travel to Zagreb - the plan was to leave for Yugoslavia in the company of Bogomil, and having arrived I would then apply for a permit to go on to Vienna and Bogomil would help me make a new start in life. A week later Bogomil visited the head of the passport service again. He told me that he had been shown my permit but that he still had to arrange a few minor things with the State Security agent. Bogomil thought that to be only a formality. It was now a few days before the 9th September; the day that the communists celebrated coming to power and everything was now postponed until after the holidays.

During the following days, everyone around me was in an ecstatic state. Galya's sister had recently married a friend of mine to whom I had introduced her. Convinced that I was now about to depart, Galya put me under pressure. Although overcome by foreboding, I married her two days before receiving my passport. Bogomil was my best man. Two days later it transpired that the State Security agent now formed an insuperable obstacle and could not be swayed. I was denied a permit and no-one could do anything about it. Galya wept and Bogomil departed for Vienna alone.

This was however not the end. On the same day, Galya informed me of her conditions for a future life together which I found completely unacceptable. We decided to separate and remain friends. It was quite obvious that our affair could not continue like that but it took months of bitterness and mutual disappointment before we finally divorced.

My sixth failure to leave the country in seven years made me feel that I had reached stalemate. Since the autumn of 1967 defection had been the most constant and important issue in my life. Everything that had happened to me in the meantime had been a consequence of my attempts to escape and I now had to pay a high price for my failure. I was thirty-two, unemployed, had no place in the country and my family relations were severely disrupted. I realized that it was necessary to move out of my grandmother's flat but I had nowhere to go. I had very little hope that I could influence the secret police agent who had blocked my final chance of leaving a country that offered me no prospect. I refused to work as an art director on the film that Galya's father was about to make; I had had enough of his influence. I felt that every day of my life in Bulgaria had been time lost.

In that state of mind in the spring of 1975 I resolved to flee in the most desperate way by illegally crossing the Yugoslav border. I was informed that the Yugoslavian authorities no longer sent back defectors from Bulgaria. One of my former classmates offered to take me across and having known that a few people had succeeded in defecting by this route I accepted his offer. In any case this seemed to be my only chance of escape.

In fact he offered me a deal: I could pay him an amount equal to three or four salary cheques. In return my former classmate would accompany me to his grandfather's village at the border and show me the road along which he said that he had walked a couple of times to the nearby Yugoslavian town of Bosilegrad, without ever having been noticed. I knew that my former classmate had a poor reputation for truthfulness but it seemed to me that the price of the deal was not terribly high.

Treklyano was a tiny village lying to the west of Sofia. His grandfather lived in an old one-storey house at the end of the village. We arrived late in the afternoon in my car and at about midnight left on foot for the border. The weather was chilly but dry and a full moon shone down upon us. We headed for a steep hill not far from the little house and after a two-hour climb arrived at the top, sweating and out of breath. Once there I was told to keep on walking in the same direction for another kilometre and then, crossing the border, I would see the lights of Bosilegrad from the top of the next hill.

I tried to do that as quickly as possible and in half an hour I reached the top of the next hill but when I looked around all I could see were yet more high dark forbidding hills in the distance. As I watched that depressing sight I realised that if I did not return before my untrustworthy guide departed for Sofia in my car I would end up in prison. Indeed when after hours of exhausting wandering I reached his grandfather's house, day was breaking.

After discussing with my guide what could have gone wrong we decided that I should give it another try. Perhaps this was because I so dearly wanted him to be right. We came back to his grandfather's house with Galya, her sister and husband. My guide and I climbed the same hill but this time he walked a few miles further with me and assured me that we had already crossed the border. Shaking with fear, he turned back and ran away leaving me alone. I walked along a narrow rough road with deep cart tracks and piles of horse dung. I had a strong feeling of foreboding. In the distance the sky was illuminated and as I climbed and reached the peak ahead I suddenly saw the explanation. Ahead of me was a nightmarish scene with a huge barbed wire concrete post fence stretching into the distance. Each post was surmounted by a dazzling searchlight. I knew that similar fences had been erected earlier along the Greek and Turkish borders and they were widely known as being impassable; even wild animals were unable to penetrate them. Immediately before me was the frontier post and I could hear dogs barking and men talking. Border guards were known for their cruelty and unquestioning obedience; they were instructed to shoot on sight anyone who attempted to cross the border and military decorations were awarded for each defector claimed.

I had no desire to die, so I turned and walked back into the maze that was closed for good behind me by the State Security agent responsible for my file. In contemplating my future once more, I had only one clear idea in my mind; I felt that I had finally stumbled on the secret of a better four-stroke engine design.

Chapter Seven
The Four-Stroke engine

At the same time that the Bulgarians were engaged in the struggle for national independence, Nikolaus Otto working in Germany invented and constructed a prototype four-stroke internal combustion engine. Otto applied for a patent that could have made him immensely rich but the inventor of the world's most widely used mechanical device had bad luck; some time before applying for his patent a Frenchman in Paris named Beau de Rochas printed a batch of a hundred copies of a booklet describing the same four-stroke cycle. Because of this, Otto spent the rest of his life ensnared in continuous legal battles while his rights to the invention were never properly protected. Thus as four-stroke engine production increased with profound effects on the course of human life, its inventor died penniless, leaving behind him what now came to be known as the Otto cycle.

Somewhat later another inventor, Rudolf Diesel, designed and built a more economical engine that was named after him. While attempting to leave Germany he died, or as some speculated was murdered, to prevent his invention from falling into enemy hands. The only engine inventor who succeeded in earning a fortune was Felix Wankel, although his rotary engine was never put into true mass production. These three are the only individuals who have successfully launched an entirely new engine concept in the automotive industry. The technology has remained largely the same as conceived by Otto more than a century ago.

The evolution of Otto's principles into the present day four-stroke engine has created a successor that appears to be completely different to the original. Huge organisations disposing of enormous budgets and with access to advanced technology have been responsible for that evolution of the essential details of the design. Today no-one expects to improve an engine's performance by revolutionising a concept in the way that Wankel did, but simply by further costly and elaborate development of the original. Nevertheless, thousands of would-be inventors continue to search for new concepts in the hope of finding that particular version which could dramatically change the course of the world's largest industry.

In 1975 I found myself in an unfavourable position compared with rival engine inventors. All things considered, to attempt to invent a new four-stroke engine at this time hardly seemed to be a suitable occupation; but I had evolved an idea that made me believe that a technological marvel might be within my reach after all.

In my concept the Otto four-stroke cycle was achieved in one revolution of the crankshaft instead of two as in the classical model. In addition valves were no longer required because the cylinders rotated in a special way in spherical sockets which opened and closed the exhaust outlets. All this took place in my imagination. My mind was busily engaged in developing a way in which my engine would be built to have advantages over the traditional design. I had a vague idea of how I should attract the interest of the motor industry to my design but still could not work out how I could leave the country in order to do that.

Every time I reached that point in my deliberations I was appalled by the realization that I might evolve a new scientific or technological concept with no means of introducing it in the West where man had already landed on the moon six years earlier.

At that time Bogomil returned to Sofia and introduced me to a friend, Nikolay Nikolov, a short dark man with a strong provincial accent who also lived in Vienna. He showed a great deal of interest in me and my problems and announced that he was eager to help me, with the claim that his contacts were much wider than Bogomil's. Who was Nikolay and how could he influence my absurd situation?

He was a violinist a little older than I who after graduating at the Conservatoire had tried to get a job abroad through the State employment agency. His application had been turned down and as he was wondering what to do next a stranger accosted him in a coffee shop with the result that after some vague discussions Nikolay and his family received permits and settled in Vienna. These influential benefactors who had made all the arrangements and whose name he could not remember obviously worked for one of the secret backbones of the regime, the intelligence service.

Besides the ominous *Sixth Chief Directorate* whose main task was to see to it that people did not get strange ideas above their station, there was another body within the enormous apparatus of the Ministry of Internal Affairs, the *Second Chief Directorate*, responsible for all subversive communist activity abroad. The activities of this body went far beyond pure intelligence work.

What was done by the personnel of the *Quiet Front*, a name amusingly used in Bulgarian literature to describe the Second Directorate's functionaries in their activities abroad will probably never be fully known. The Bulgarian secret services were in fact a direct extension of the Soviet system; their tasks and their personnel enjoyed the highest standing in the country. Stalin had constantly striven to turn that branch of the KGB into the most powerful organisation of its kind in the world. Its activities included everything that made it an efficient instrument of communist politics; the recruitment of spies, the theft of nuclear and technological secrets, the support of dictators, terrorists and assassins.

Nikolay seemed to have been recruited by that invisible organisation in exchange for his permit to work abroad. Possibly his assignment was to establish certain business activities and send part of the profits to his benefactors. Although hardly intelligent, he was certainly ambitious to succeed in his task. I reached these conclusions after a few lengthy discussions with Nikolay. Bogomil was always present and probably he also worked for those services as an informer which was why he was allowed to repair violins in Vienna.

In the end Nikolay came up with a proposal. He undertook to arrange a passport for me to go to Vienna on the condition that he would receive half of my income once I took out a patent and launched my invention in the West. This was something for me to consider. I did not like the proposal or Nikolay and least of all his benefactors who did not enjoy the reputation of sympathetic and considerate people.

But what choice did I have? Having failed to cross the Yugoslavian border I tried once more to defect; this time by boarding a ship sailing between Varna and Istanbul across the Black Sea. This was my ninth attempt to defect in the last eight years and I quickly realised that my plan was bound to fail. There seemed to be nothing new left to me to try and during that period my life seemed to fall completely apart.

I tried to earn my living as an artist but the income was small and I saw myself getting into constant debt. Almost every day I visited my son Viktor, only to realize how unable I

The Four-Stroke engine

was to help his grandfather who looked after him and who besides had personal troubles in his relationship with Rositsa.

My grandmother, now seventy-five, complained about my erratic presence in her flat. My brother was quick to fill the gap and he and his family moved in - he even ensured that grandmother gave him the bigger car and that the white Renault 8 that I had driven as a student was returned to me. After a painful period trying to settle down I returned to the old attic without being able to rely on my parents for help.

No-one seemed to understand how I could have descended to such a poor state. As my attempts to defect were followed and punished I did not dare to discuss my plans and all the other subjects that kept my mind alive and this was not easy.

Communism profoundly changed human nature in the countries where it held sway. As the Berlin Wall came down many people believed that the differences that the collapsing system had revealed would soon vanish. Years later however the Wall was still present in their minds, dividing the German nation into two groups of completely different people. These same changes were all the more profound in Bulgaria; there the making of the *new man* as the communisation of the individual was developed was yet further beyond the situation in any other East European country.

Many believed that the system was sensible and their primitive fanaticism would never submit to reasonable argument. They easily took in their stride the abyss between the concept of justice and the killings and repression of millions. If things went wrong this must all be due to the fault of individuals or to influences from abroad.

Many communists however were simply shrewd social climbers who believed only in having the power and the privileges that went with it. Such people represented a majority in the huge bureaucratic apparatus and to them human values were one of those empty slogans issued by the Party; whoever held power was in the right and those who refused to obey must be enemies. To safeguard their own position such people were ready to do anything and often did.

The rest of the population was simply intimidated and held in subservience. Any sign of conflict with the communist system could ruin one's whole life and as a result at least in public no-one dared contest anything. The area beyond what was considered to be established communist philosophy was forbidden territory.

A small group of people failed to comply with those standards and under an article in the criminal code on *seditious campaigning and propaganda* they risked a prison sentence of several years because of their anti-socialist statements and conduct. In the language of the state security that meant `discontent with the socialist system, applauding the Western way of living, listening to and discussing the broadcasts of subversive radio stations, reading or writing text advocating anti-socialist views, defaming communist ideas, authorities and countries, telling jokes and disseminating decadence through music and other art forms'.

The most severe punishment was reserved for those who had the temerity to contact others sharing their views - they would be brutally repressed under another law providing Draconian measures to combat anything that could be identified as *movements and groups in opposition*.

Those classified as politically unreliable lost their jobs and risked being sent into internal exile or to a labour camp. Often they would be *immunised* by a process involving continual threats interspersed with savage beating. The object of this was to harass them until they abandoned all human dignity and were reduced to a miserable shadow of their former self.　This was of course achieved by means of institutionalised cruelty totally unconnected with a legal process based on the observance of morality.　Reportedly, some of those who refused to give in to the process would be left to the tender mercy of other, psychotic, inmates; frequently resulting in death.

The authorities boasted that there remained not a vestige of opposition, dissidence or revolt in Bulgaria unlike the other communist countries, including the Soviet Union.

My desperate desire to defect had brought me to the point at which I had to make a choice between being shot by a frontier guard or being cast into prison.　What else could I look forward to if unable to keep my views to myself?　When I considered this impasse, I understood that I could not ignore Nikolay's proposal. He asked nothing of me that might bring me into contact with his anonymous benefactors.　If I could buy my freedom with money earned in the future I was prepared to do that without regret.　It seemed to me at the time that I could even tolerate having one of my hands cut off if that were necessary.

So one day at the end of the summer of 1975 I reached a verbal agreement with Nikolay.　He undertook to provide me with a permit in exchange for half the royalties from my four-stroke internal combustion engine.　Bogomil stood as witness to the agreement.

As agreed I then applied for a permit to travel to Vienna in response to an invitation sent to me by Nikolay.　Before leaving he asked me for documentation that would give him an idea of my potential.　I gave him a copy of my paper on quantum mechanics and photographs of some of my designs.　None of that was secret but the very thought that the intelligence services would now see my work made me feel uneasy.

To keep my side of the bargain I began work on the drawings of my future four-stroke engine.　I liked to linger over my drawing-board late at night, listening to music with a cup of coffee and a cigarette.　My mind would wander to a wide range of subjects before again concentrating on the sheet before me.　It is always a long route from the general concept of an engine to the detailed drawing of each individual component.　I moved forward a step at a time, constantly modifying and improving every detail as I progressed.

Again I persuaded my former classmate Branimir to cooperate with me on the project just as we had on our failed design for a rotary engine.　We did not tell the Institute of Inventions on this occasion however.　I made a deal with Branimir to estimate the value of his cooperation in the enterprise so that I could reward him once I had managed to go abroad.　He agreed but we both appreciated that the practical outcome of that project was still very uncertain and the most likely revenue from it would be the pleasure given by the work itself.

Working on the engine did indeed give us great enjoyment.　Late in the afternoon Branimir would come to my grandmother's or to Galya's flat and we would sit at the drawing-board to spend hours in the fantasy world of imaginary engines.　Sometimes we would become completely carried away in our discussion of the engine, its parts and all about it; often until dawn.　Branimir would lie on the sofa for a couple of hours and go back to his office in the morning while the engine acquired an increasingly distinctive form on the rather smudgy drawing.

Branimir suffered from a difficult marriage.　His wife, a dominant down-to-earth and beautiful woman made no secret of her lack of respect for him.　She constantly harassed him by quoting him the example of more successful individuals in unfavourable comparison.　Branimir was not like them.　He was sensitive and considerate and felt ill at ease about his humble career as an engineer.　One day the worm turned and his usual passive tolerance collapsed under an outburst of rage.　He left his wife, hired an attic barely large

The Four-Stroke engine

enough to accommodate a bed and lived there the life of a stoic barely surviving on his tiny salary.

Branimir and I had a strong bond of understanding. We both felt unsuited to live within the communist system. At the end of the year Branimir resigned from our joint project explaining that he had become involved with a girl and intended to marry her. Some years later he defected to the West while on an overseas business trip. He tried to make a living in Belgium and later moved on to the United States. I never heard anything further from him. His departure was painful to me and he has always remained in my memory.

The drawings of the engine and a small wooden drawing-board were my constant companions wherever I went. They finally ended up with me in the tiny attic that I occupied during my years at the academy. I returned after four years of unsuccessful endeavours to leave the country, two failed marriages and once more without employment. My total achievements so far amounted to an article on theoretical physics launching the basis of a new theory and the concept of an engine recorded in an unfinished drawing; neither of which offered any great hope for the near future.

My parents were deeply concerned about me but I did not wish to trouble them with my personal problems. Some years previously my father had undergone a serious operation for cancer. The consequences of this were painful but he could not yet afford to retire. My sister was still a student. I felt I was a burden to them all and did my best not to worry them by trying to manage alone in the poorly-furnished attic. Under those circumstances my deal with Nikolay appeared to be my only ray of hope. Within me I had serious doubts about its chances of success and despite all my efforts at optimism I had a deep premonition about Nikolay, which was justified by events. I should have received an answer from the passport department months previously.

Nikolay returned to Sofia and after many discussions confronted me with new conditions that took me by surprise. Claiming that there was a general lack of confidence, he insisted that he could only vouch for me by providing evidence to the authorities that I could be trusted to keep my side of the bargain. I was somewhat curious to know what kind of evidence this would require. It turned out to be the drawings of my engine.

I was in a weak position to bargain but I asked Nikolay why he needed the drawings if he was now swearing that he would not show them to anyone. Nikolay had no understanding of engine construction and would be unable to understand the value of the drawings as evidence of my potential. But he would not allow argument, claiming that he trusted me in the deal and I now had to prove that I trusted him too by giving him the drawings.

This seemed illogical and that night as I lay on the hard creaking bed in the attic I kept thinking about what I should do. Under the poorly insulated roof heated by the rays of the sun, the air was oppressive and swarms of mosquitoes kept me awake.

Chain-smoking one cigarette after another, I came to appreciate that I was not in a situation where logical behaviour was important. So I reached the simple conclusion that it mattered not what Nikolay intended to do with my drawings if by giving them to him I could leave the country.

On the following day I gave Nikolay a copy of the still incomplete design and made him promise that he would not show it to anyone without prior consultation. Bogomil was present too. Soon after they left my application for a permit was again rejected. Nikolay seemed very surprised when I called him and hurried to say that he would look into matters.

Very little happened before the beginning of the next year. At the age of thirty-three I felt that I inhabited a nightmare world from which I desperately wished to escape.

During the winter I spent many more lonely hours in the attic working on the engine. Finally I had a complete draft of an application for a patent and a precise set of drawings that seemed to me to offer a good basis for building a prototype. My belief in the engine design was extremely strong. I am not sure that it was based entirely on reason since inventors tend to be fanatical rather than reasonable individuals. Perhaps an unquestioning belief by the inventor in a new idea is essential to launch it successfully.

I wondered what I should do with my invention if I was unable to leave the country. Despite its endorsement of Lenin's concept of the state ownership of inventions, Bulgaria had signed the Paris Convention on industrial ownership. At least theoretically an inventor could apply for a private patent to safeguard his copyright, yet this was never done. On first contact with the bureaucrats at the Institute of Inventions applicants were warned to not even think of applying for a private patent. No-one was anxious to cross the authorities and inventors therefore applied for an *author's certificate* which voluntarily relinquished all copyright to the Bulgarian state. In any case there was little point in issuing a private patent since private entrepreneurship did not exist and was moreover considered reprehensible. There was another major obstacle: international patent protection was an expensive procedure that halted even the wildest dreams of Bulgarian inventors seeking financial success.

With all this in mind I realized that I could do little with my engine in Bulgaria. However while thinking of how copyright was formally recognized but yet rudely violated, I became aware of a new idea taking shape in my mind.

The absolute intolerance of any form of dissent was universal. All writers were obliged to publicly renounce Solzhenitsyn's work as `slanderous'. One, who had not yet read Solzhenitsyn's work, refused to do so because of his unfamiliarity with it. He was immediately expelled from the Writer's Union and consequently was unable to continue his chosen profession. The hysterical tone of the press and paranoid demonstrations of faithful conformity at public gatherings demonstrated that the regime was anxious to prevent any sign of dissent from reaching the outside world.

I asked myself whether I could profit from these obsessions by confronting the State Security with a choice: either allow me to go abroad or admit to the outside world that there was real protest in the country. By signing the Helsinki Conference documents, the Bulgarian authorities had formally declared their willingness to respect human rights; I thought that I could use that as an argument to permit me to emigrate.

This seemed a desperately hazardous plan but it might be my only chance of success. My plan seemed logical enough to me but as I understood later, was utterly naive. I was now a lonely and isolated man who had reached the point at which conformity with the communist system seemed totally out of the question. No one of course would dream of taking the enormous risk of lending support to my protest.

As if to make matters worse my emotional life had entered a new dark period. My marriage to Galya lasted only a couple of months and that only because we were not able to get divorced immediately after our wedding as we had agreed, because the legal process was still continuing. I had not expected that it would be so difficult to part from her and was much displeased with myself because of the way in which I had handled the affair.

The girls who had been interested in me in earlier years now seemed to have disappeared. If by any chance I met a girl I was either totally obsessed with my

The Four-Stroke engine

attempts to defect or felt so confused that I failed to take up the challenge of entering into a relationship.

During the summer I had gone to Varna in an attempt to defect by boarding a Black Sea steamer. Walking in the street I saw a beautiful girl coming towards me. Her long brown hair shone in the sun. The nearer she came the more desperately beautiful she seemed to me. An aircraft flew low over the city and I stopped and looked up at it. She put down her heavy bag on the pavement and looked too. We both followed the plane until it disappeared and then our eyes met. She said something to me in Italian and then in English. I realized that I was lost in the way that I had always dreamed about. I knew that I had to go with her. I forced myself not to do so, realizing how desperately weak I was and how difficult it would be to continue with my attempt to board the ship. As she turned and walked away from me I felt an urge to run after her. My intuition told me that I had just lost something I would probably never find again.

I spent the wet winter of 1976 a lonely man with leaking shoes and an old pair of jeans in the cold dirty attic among heaps of paper lying on the floor. In February I decided to abandon the deal with Nikolay. I telephoned him and said that I intended to apply for a patent in Sofia and expected him to send back the article, photographs and the drawings. Some of the photographs that I had given him were the only copies that I had.

Nikolay explained to me he could not possibly do that as he had already filed for a patent on his and my behalf. As to my passport, that could obviously not be arranged for the time being.

Things began to look rather unpleasant.

In the past six months of waiting for a result I kept thinking that under the worst circumstances Nikolay would fail to arrange a permit and that would leave me to face the fact that emigration was simply out of the question. I felt that I was resigned to that prospect. Rather naively I never even imagined that Nikolay might blackmail me if anything went wrong. It seemed to me that that had just happened and I had no idea of what to do next. I must act quickly however, otherwise I could be in for more trouble.

Obviously Nikolay had contacts with the secret service. On one occasion when held up by the traffic police in Sofia because of a minor offence he treated the officer with contempt and arrogance in a manner quite unthinkable for the general public. It seemed that he was even more arrogant now; no-one would dare to do what he claimed that he had done. Had he really filed for a patent? Was there a secret service agent involved in this transaction? What did Nikolay mean by telling me all that?

I found it difficult to answer those questions. Obviously Nikolay was dishonest and dangerous and I could not influence his behaviour simply by talking to him on the telephone. In fact I was being subjected to straightforward blackmail. Nikolay was absolutely sure that because I would never dare contact his benefactors he could force me into accepting whatever it was that he intended to do with my invention. However, he was mistaken.

During a couple of sleepless nights I prepared the draft and the drawings of the engine with the intention of applying for a patent at the Institute of Inventions. I wrote a short appeal in support of my rights including the right to travel and referred to the Helsinki Declaration. I enclosed copies of my appeal, the draft for a patent application and the drawings in two envelopes that I gave to Nina who had remained my good friend ever since she had seen me off on my first attempt to leave the country over nine years ago. I asked her to find the way to take them to some of the Western embassies in Sofia in case I might disappear or be arrested in the next few days.

She agreed although I warned her that she was running a considerable risk. Early on the morning of the 24th February 1976 I filed for a private patent at the Institute of Inventions. My application shocked the officials who had never experienced a similar act of defiance. I was obliged to pay a truly outrageous fee.

Next I went to the reception room at the Ministry of the Interior and insisted on speaking to whoever was in charge of crime involving intelligence personnel. The official was surprised too but asked me to sit and wait. Soon a young athletic-looking man in a dark suit entered and asked me for a summary of my story. He wrote down a couple of names and left saying that he had to check up a few things. I waited for half an hour and then the young man returned to introduce himself as Evgeniev and asked me into a small office to discuss the matter further.

Our conversation lasted about an hour and in the end he advised me not to mention the matter to anyone nor to return to the Ministry but to wait for him to contact me on the following day. Walking in the narrow street from the Ministry to my home, I felt ready to exchange my future life for any other destiny; I was deeply disturbed by the mysterious scenario that was now unfolding before me.

Chapter Eight
Vocation: Bastard

On the following day, Evgeniev took me to a garage where the exalted members of the communist *nomenclatura's* limousines, square-styled black Chaikas, were kept. The head of the garage showed interest in my invention and for the first time I was able to demonstrate how the engine worked and its potential advantages using my drawings and a small scale-model built of Meccano. As a mechanic, he was able to quickly grasp the idea and showed enthusiasm for it.

A long period of silence followed until one day Evgeniev telephoned to inform me that in future I would be approached by a different official.

Early one afternoon when I was alone in my parents' flat the doorbell rang and I opened the front door to a tall balding young man with a dark complexion and nervous smile who flashed his official identity card under my nose. I invited him to come in and thus at last met Georgi Gaydarov, the State Security officer who had been responsible for my file during the last few years. There right in front of me stood the man who on four occasions had flatly refused to allow me to travel abroad and was therefore the root cause of all my present problems.

Gaydarov, a few years younger than I, seemed excited and restless but was rather overfriendly and inquisitive. He told me that he had lived and studied in Belgium where his parents were posted presumably to work at the Bulgarian embassy in Brussels. He had a marked aversion to the West; said that life there was disgustingly comfortable but I suspected that his dislike was more based on the depressing isolation in which he would have found himself abroad.

The State Security organisation chose its officers from among the core of ambitious and fanatical young men able to offer an impeccable communist background. Most of them were then trained at a special State Security school located in what had once been the Sofia American college at the foot of the Vitosha mountain. Most of these young men lived a life dreaming that they would one day become the embodiment of the most popular character stereotyped in Bulgarian literature of the time; the brave intelligence officer battling with the CIA amidst capitalist depravity and lechery. Many of them were obsessed by that romantic ideal and among those whose applications to join the organisation were rejected, cases of nervous breakdown and depression were reported.

In reality these were the people trained to create the dark side of the communist system. When communism finally fell, the general public for the first time learned about the extent and universality of the omnipotent secret services throughout Eastern Europe. Their monstrous methods of repression and violence, threat and manipulation were at last revealed and it became clear that they were prepared to destroy lives in order to maintain the system and to cruelly suppress every attempt to reject official dogma. Naturally all those working for the secret services were merely a cog within a huge repressive machine far more terrifying than Kafkaesque and Orwellian fiction.

At this time however I only had a vague idea of Gaydarov's responsibilities. Because he was in charge of my file that meant that he knew everything about me - all the gossip and slander - and had so far successfully thwarted all my plans to flee the country. He asked me about my invention and my difficulties with Nikolay. He showed a keen interest in everything to do with me and my engine although I expected that he knew it already and I was therefore eager to find out what he was actually trying to achieve. After a few weeks of meetings and discussions in a variety of cafés I thought that I knew what he was after.

The secret service must have understood the importance of my engine, otherwise they would never have sent Gaydarov to visit me. Moreover his interest demonstrated that Nikolay in fact had cooperated with a member of the intelligence service although it was not clear to what extent that other person had been involved in the patent application process. As intelligence officers were extremely influential and above the law, Nikolay felt safe to attempt to blackmail me because he was certain that I would not be in a position to do anything about it. Nikolay continued to claim that he had filed for a patent long before my application and if I had not reacted I would have been continually blackmailed.

I also came to understand that someone high in the secret service hierarchy, probably even a deputy minister in charge of the intelligence services, had overseen my case and had protected my interests continuously. This would explain why Gaydarov's attitude to me was friendly.

Eventually I was summoned to the police department of the Lenin district where I lived and where Gaydarov was based. I was shown into the office of the district head of state security, Colonel Christozko Uzunov. Colonel Uzunov would never have got far if his physical appearance was all that mattered. Little mercy could be expected from this puffy face with slit eyes and deep wrinkles. His manner and vocabulary only emphasised that unfortunate impression. Once a mere peasant, Uzunov had been active in the Communist Resistance and had probably based his career on liquidating enemies of the regime. The fact that he had reached such an elevated rank at Sofia's central district police authority meant that he was not known for treating sympathetically those classified as enemies of the Party.

During our conversation a tall white-haired and blue-eyed man of about fifty came into Uzunov's office without introducing himself. At his arrival I immediately sensed a heightened note of respect in Uzunov's voice as the man's authority filled the room. The new arrival did not take part in our conversation but merely sat and listened carefully. Finally he asked me how Nikolay would respond if we were to meet privately.

I never learned the name of that mysterious man but through the window I could see a black Chaika waiting for him and I guessed that this was my hidden protector. I never met him again.

Soon after that meeting Gaydarov informed me that Nikolay would come to Sofia and I was expected to meet him to discuss the matter. Nikolay visited me in my attic. His visit was brief and I asked him why he had not kept his part of the bargain and how he could possibly have filed for a patent without my consent. He was as rudely impertinent as ever; his only argument was that in Bulgaria I could do very little with my invention. At this I reminded him that our bargain was only valid if he could arrange for me to leave the country and that he had given me his word that he would make no use of the drawings that he had requested as evidence.

Nikolay was not in the least concerned about having broken his bond to me. There was little more to say and I asked him to leave. He was simply an imposter and later I learned that his passport had been confiscated and that he had been banned from leaving the country on regular business. A year later however he succeeded in emigrating and rejoined his wife and daughter in Vienna.

The affair ended with the final conversation with Gaydarov who assured me that Nikolay would never trouble me again and I could forget all about him. He added that I was now free to file for a patent in my name.

Although it was true that Nikolay would cause me no further difficulty, I had now fallen into the hands of the guardians of the ideology, who immediately prevented me from succeeding in my tenth attempt in nine years to leave the country. The agents of the secret service had now come out of the shadows and in personal talks intended to explore my projects, my way of life and views, now had far greater influence over me. The officers of the secret service were omnipotent and able to interfere in and determine the destiny of any mortal outside the ruling hierarchy.

At our meetings Gaydarov made no secret of the fact that it was he who had refused to allow me to emigrate in recent years. He disagreed totally with my views and never neglected to point out that I refused absolutely to accept the basic communist ideology while others although demonstrating their discontent still remained true to communism. In 1974 he had thwarted Bogomil's attempt to obtain a permit for me to travel abroad, thus indirectly causing the failure of my second marriage. He only did this because he wished to demonstrate that he was more important than Galya's father, the film producer Borislav Sharaliev, a colonel in the State Security himself. Gaydarov took intense pleasure in letting fall during our conversations how important he was. Sometimes he would erupt in uncontrollable laughter that suddenly turned into abject whining.

This time however things were different. Recognizing the potential importance of my invention, State Security was now seriously interested in my fate. A note had been made of my qualities as an inventor and scientist in the files of the State Security and this newfound reputation would now follow me during the next fourteen years before I could finally leave Bulgaria.

On one occasion Gaydarov suggested that I could work at a secret scientific institute that would give me all that I needed to carry out my experiments. He implied that people of my kind could be promoted to the rank of general during the scientific research programme. This was not in any sense a passing remark. The fact that senior State Security officers were openly interested in me formed an indisputable invitation to join them in the secret service. This was a prospect that aroused no enthusiasm in me.

On my meeting with Gaydarov I took the opportunity to raise the question of my possible emigration. He immediately warned me that any attempt on my part to publicise my objections to the regime would be secretly and firmly suppressed. I was later informed that not a single one of those Bulgarians who had contacted Western embassies in an attempt to defect had subsequently been allowed to leave the country and they had all been persecuted for their resistance. Gaydarov emphasised that I would never be permitted to work abroad on my invention. If I continued to take this line I would be forced to join the intelligence service where any infringement of the rules would be punished with a bullet.

At the end of spring 1976 I had filed for a patent on a four-stroke engine but was still unemployed and had no prospects for the future. A patent application would secure international protection of my rights over the invention for a year but after that I would have to apply for a patent abroad and this was a costly procedure. At this time I had to deal with the administration of the Institute for Inventions and there remained many unknown factors because this was the first private patent ever issued in Bulgaria under the Communist Government. Even if I were to succeed in obtaining my patent I was still faced by a large problem: the Bulgarian State had the monopoly of trade with foreign companies and as a private citizen I had no right to contact anyone with a business offer. The only hope that I had was to attract the attention of the automotive industry by publishing an article on my engine together with a drawing and description amounting to some ten pages.

This seemed a rather poor way to introduce a new engine, yet I believed absolutely in my success although I did not have the vaguest idea of how I could achieve it. Except for the functionaries of the secret service, very few people in Sofia believed that working on my engine would make any sense at all. It seemed beyond the question to ever attain the accepted levels of Western technology and most people in the East lived under an inferiority complex about such things. Under those circumstances the very concept of a new engine would only provoke disbelief and scepticism. I was often faced by derision from those I knew including the unimaginative family of my second ex-wife.

During recent months I had spent much time with my friend Doctor Lyuben Kanov, a clinical psychiatrist. Lyubo was a tall man with easy manners and a ridiculous sense of humour. He was intelligent and balanced and attracted the attention of all with his strong personality which shone in any company. However, behind his superficial stability Lyubo was as obsessed with the idea of defecting as I and it was his idea to go to Varna and take a steamer bound for Istanbul. This wasn't much of an idea perhaps but we gave it a try.

Lyubo's younger brother, a design student, had successfully emigrated to Canada a few years earlier. This meant that Lyubo had not the slightest chance of ever travelling abroad himself; the revenge of the secret service had placed him in the same desperate position that I occupied. But although he tried so hard to be careful and to avoid any misdemeanour in the eyes of the State he was nevertheless frequently depressed because of his inability to leave Bulgaria. He was a gifted storyteller and in the written word expressed doubt as to whether his life made any sense at all.

Except for Lyubo there were few people with whom I could share my problems. In the last strenuous months of waiting hopelessly for a permit and because of this the investigation into my unsuccessful deal with Nikolay, I had lost touch with reality. I seemed to be in free fall; was unemployed and had few friends. It was constantly difficult to make ends meet and often grandmother had to help me out to avoid disaster.

It was in those days of seeming weightlessness that I met Todor (Tosho) Tolev, a fair-haired delightful giant from Trebich, a village near Sofia. Tosho was anything but shy, a full-blooded Shopp bursting with energy and ready to chat with any stranger he met. This is exactly what Tosho did when he met me in a café one day and became a friend who stuck with me for a long time.

Tosho had graduated in mechanical engineering but openly admitted that he had achieved this success thanks to generous bribes paid by his father to his professors. This was the way that he generally got along in life and I have to admit that it was a successful system. He had a job normally with a research centre where he would turn up for a couple of minutes each day. He spent the rest of his time at the Defence Ministry's sports club playing chess or billiards at which he was quite good. He often played for money and said that this routine helped him to relax.

Very soon Tosho won my friendship with his generous open-hearted nature and his sympathy for my problems. He spent most of his free time with me helping in any way he could.

Vocation: Bastard

He was a very unselfish man indeed and after visiting my tiny attic he took me to the small flat where he lived with his wife and daughter and promptly insisted that I should move in. Beside this he was willing to undertake all kinds of small favours and as I had to type my letters for the patent application he offered to lend me a typewriter from his office.

Late one afternoon we drove to Tosho's office in his green Lada. At the entrance we ran into Georgi Gaydarov who left in an embarrassed hurry. This chance encounter brought me to a horrifying conclusion; State Security now had me under 24-hour surveillance. Gaydarov had been sent to investigate Tosho because of his contacts with me. He had just spoken to the personnel manager responsible for all information about staff and the timing of the visit made it clear that it had been carefully planned because Tosho was never to be found at his office late in the afternoon.

I explained to Tosho why it was that Gaydarov was interested in me and urged him to no longer run the risk of being observed trying to give help. However he would not listen and beside having a stubborn nature himself he had relatives working for the State Security who had protected him previously. They had shielded him from trouble before and he felt quite safe under their protection.

During those years nothing was ever published or generally known about the specific methods of the invisible State Security system. Although so many people worked for it, all the information concerning its activities was classified. No-one was free to discuss the methods used by the State Security and those who were in any way aware would avoid making any comment or observation.

When I realized that I was being kept under surveillance I was in fact unaware of what this really meant.

The agents of State Security could shadow anyone without provoking suspicion. In order to instigate an investigation into a person it was sufficient to send incriminating information or merely a report claiming that a fellow citizen was in some way involved in *ideological subversion*. All those who resisted the communist dogma on life were persecuted. Those investigated were watched closely by all possible means. This could imply telephone tapping, the use of bugging devices in their home, secret house searches and the recruitment of friends and relatives as informers. It could mean gross interference in all institutions and organisations throughout the country. The investigation could continue for months and assume monstrous dimensions. No cost or human resource would be spared if the

information gained proved that the guardians of ideological purity indeed had well-founded suspicions. The process of harassment would usually end with forceful repression.

Investigation by State Security enjoyed the highest priority and no-one would be allowed to help or even to put in a good word to support the person being `worked upon'. As a result of general corruption it could be arranged that citizens were found not guilty on charges of murder, theft or other crimes but there was no mercy at all for those sinning against *communist ideology* and no one dared offer any assistance to the unfortunate suspect.

No one - whether political dissident or even an ancient communist from the days of the Resistance - would be forgiven for rejecting the accepted ideology. Anyone who was being worked upon could only seek mercy by kneeling before the immortal mummy of Lenin or for that matter Zhivkov, his Bulgarian substitute.

In that atmosphere of suspicion, the officers of State Security watched most vigorously of all over the ideological purity and zeal of their own colleagues. In their endeavour to demonstrate their total devotion they would sometimes treat their helpless victims with feral ferocity. In their pursuit of a brilliant career, secret service agents would often exaggerate or even invent *ideological crimes* and signs of hostile activity in desperately frustrated citizens unable to maintain the false appearance of conformity amid the hypocrisy and denunciation everywhere around.

Georgi Gaydarov was a man of many complexes but also of great ambition. He dreamed constantly of gaining even greater power and that became obvious in our discussions. On one occasion he even complained to me about the stupidity of his bosses and the inadequacy of his salary.

It was obvious that Gaydarov expected me to be grateful to him for everything that had happened to me during recent years. He gave the impression of being hurt by my refusal to cooperate with the secret service and the way in which I had turned down his offer of friendship. Some of the unpleasant remarks that I had made about him were brought to his notice and had made him furious. The fact that a high-ranking official had taken me under his wing persuaded Gaydarov to prove that despite my invention I was an enemy class and that he was correct in his conclusions about me. In any case it was easy for Gaydarov to begin working on me; my unprecedented application for a private patent gave him a good excuse. Possibly he imagined that he stood a fair chance of impressing his superiors by working on a case that had attracted the attention of the highest officials.

Even after I realized that I was being shadowed it still did not occur to me that my conversations would be recorded, my attic and my parents' flat secretly searched and all those in my circle investigated.

In desperation resulting from my last failure to escape, I clung like a drowning man to a straw, imagining that my engine would attract the attention of foreign companies. To contemplate the harmony and beauty of the imaginary components of my engine was the only real pleasure to me amid the nightmare of reality.

My engine resembled an octagonal star, in the points of which were mounted the spherical sockets for the cylinders. But that star seemed to give no hope to my invention and those around me.

Tosho's brother worked for the Bulgarian Transport Monopoly and travelled all over Europe. The idea of crossing the border hidden in his heavy truck came to me spontaneously; I told myself that whatever happened, it could never be worse than to endure the present situation. I shared my idea with Lyubo Kanov, who sunk yet further into his depressed and sceptical moods.

One night Tosho and I examined a heavy truck covered with thick canvas sheeting. For once Tosho's natural courage seemed to desert him and he said that he would be in deep trouble if I were to hide in the truck. I remembered something that Tosho had once told me - as a boy he had once wagered that he could climb a pylon. The electrical current had flung him to the ground and he had broken his legs.

After a brief moment of reflection I abandoned my eleventh attempt to escape. Instead Tosho and I went to the seaside for a short holiday. I needed rest from the despair of reality and my continuing fanciful plans for defection.

On the road to Sozopol two young French girls thumbed a lift. We stopped Tosho's Lada to pick them up. Marion, a tall slender dark-haired Parisienne was interested in me and I liked her too but I had to suppress my urge to ask her to lend me her passport so that I could attempt to cross the border with it. In the evening I had to drag Tosho away from them and as we travelled further I told him about my obsession with Marion's passport.

The inner desire to leave the country had taken a painfully firm hold on me and never left me in peace for a single moment. Throughout day and night I continually thought of all possible and impossible ways to defect but my instinct told me that an invisible enemy was closing in around me.

My instincts had not misled me. On one occasion Tosho had accurately repeated something that a relative of his had said about me; these comments were intended to reach me. The man worked for the Sixth Department of State Security and had commented on something I had said on the telephone on the previous day. It was not hard to understand the message and to realize the appalling nature of my situation.

For months I had openly discussed anything I thought about with friends on the telephone or in private conversations. I mentioned my plans to get out of the country and talked about everything that had happened. All the time, day in; day out, my comments, thoughts and reactions had been recorded. Now they were in the hands of Gaydarov and his bosses who could reproduce anything I had said with greater precision than I could remember it.

It was easy to conclude that there was not even the faintest chance to leave the country in view of the way that I was kept under surveillance. At the moment however, I wished to know what it was that State Security intended to do with me.

I decided to discuss the matter openly with Gaydarov. In the autumn we met in a small room at the police department of the Lenin district in Sofia. He seemed very pleased with himself and commented openly about the extensive information that he had amassed by spying on me. Gaydarov arrogantly mentioned that neither heavy trucks nor Marion's passport would help me get out of the country. If I had tried any of those possibilities we would have met much earlier. He was so well informed about all my plans for defection - even those I had forgotten about long ago. Without concealing his deep satisfaction, Gaydarov remarked on the subjects that I had not even considered at all.

During the sleepless nights of recent months I had begun to work on a story about all that had happened to me. I referred to those spying on me as intellectual midgets. In my story Gaydarov could read my thoughts with the help of a special electronic device. Once he was especially pleased to record my thought that communism was a higher form of organised crime. In parenthesis I commented on the use of the phrase `a higher form' as typical Marxist jargon making it easier for my investigators to understand.

Gaydarov had no need of a device to read my thoughts since he had just read and copied my text while searching through my attic. The consequences of this did not seem pleasant but still I could not help laughing at the very thought of Gaydarov reading my comments about him.

To have written text like mine was at that time punished mercilessly. I could have been arrested immediately and sent to prison purely because of that original material left in my room. Immediately Gaydarov and Colonel Uzunov used their consummate skill in such matters to blackmail me. They faced me with a brutal choice: I could either write down a confession that they would dictate to me or I would be arrested and agents sent to collect the text from my attic room.

This investigation of me would put others at risk, too. I explained to Lyubo Kanov and a couple of friends I had seen in the last month that I was being watched and suggested that they should cease contact with me. They all agreed to do this but I still worried about them.

Tosho was the only one to break the complete isolation in which I found myself as a result of the State Security operation. He simply refused to abandon me. He believed that his relatives working for the State Security of whom one was a general, would protect him. Tosho sympathised with me and took my side but nevertheless on one occasion asked me not to confide in him because he did not wish to betray me in case he might be forced to do so.

In this situation the only flicker of optimism was my continuing belief in my engine invention. Each night before falling asleep I thought over time and time again every part of the engine in my search for ways to improve it. In reality the real problems that I had to face were very little to do with the mechanical parts that I refined and assembled in my mind. The private patent application met resistance from the very first expert dealing with the matter and now I was at war with the bureaucracy of the Institute of Inventions. Despite the threat from having clashed with socialist standards and showing disrespect for Lenin, my application could not be turned down on the grounds of prior art or technical imperfection.

By the end of the year I worried about the scant progress made with my patent application. I also worried about comments made to me by Tosho after meeting his influential relatives. Tosho looked ill-at-ease and concerned; he recommended me to make my invention public and announce that Western observers would be told about it if anything happened to me. My conclusion from this was that the secret service had been discussing a possible arranged disappearance of my application. Would I too disappear as part of the same plot?

At last however on 23rd December 1976, my private patent for a four-stroke internal combustion engine was registered with the authorities. On the same day I was given permission to file for a patent abroad at my own expense. As far as I know that was the first time a private patent had ever been issued to a Bulgarian inventor in his own country.

At the beginning of the new year an application for a patent was filed on my behalf in most countries with a domestic automotive industry. The Institute for Inventions was put in charge of the application and I was forced to pay the cost amounting to $5000 within the year. At that time the sum was equal to ten years' salary. Naturally enough $5000 was as out of my reach as five million. I was unemployed and the odd jobs I did such as decorating or sign-writing had become very infrequent. My daily expenses were covered by my grandmother and my parents and even buying a pair of shoes was a seemingly insuperable problem. I was thirty-three years old. The State Security's investigation had made it quite impossible for me to have friends and I lived in complete isolation in my tiny shabby attic. To escape from that situation, I was relying solely on the patent application that had been sent across the border to a world beyond my reach. This was not just optimism.

By now the rotary engine of Felix Wankel which had been launched on 23rd November 1959 was nearing the end of its twenty-year history in the public eye. It had infected me with inventor's virus and had fired the imagination of many others. Wankel's engine was licensed to many concerns worldwide; it was improved, notably by the German company NSU after extensive research, and had been installed in several thousand cars with plans for mass production under way. But because the largest world car manufacturer, General Motors, had abandoned the idea of using it, the classical poppet valve four-stroke engine was still the only type used in motor cars. Examination of the Wankel design had incurred huge expense by the licensees and the fact that the expected revolution had failed to materialise enhanced the sceptical reaction to all types of new engine design. It was therefore unlikely that my patent application would attract attention.

The working of my engine design was not easy to follow and besides, special precision machine tools were required to manufacture the spherical parts. Hardly anyone could be expected to invest in its development without a virtual guarantee of profit. I myself had no illusions about the possibility of manufacturing the engine in Bulgaria and I still remembered the failure of another project in Varna. My application would not be published until August and even if anyone then was interested I could not imagine how that might change my personal situation.

Vocation: Bastard

In fact things could only become worse. The State Security forces had gone to great expense in keeping me under surveillance for an entire year and would hardly be prepared to sit back and watch to see if a foreign company might be willing to invest in my work. I was now still under surveillance and a translator I knew was investigated by State Security purely because I had asked him to help me with the translation of my application. Tosho told me that his well-informed relatives had suggested that a prototype of my engine had been constructed in the Soviet Union but had failed at the first test. In any case it was not easy to imagine the profitability that a private patent on my invention might bring. It was most likely to cost me a fortune.

One morning Tosho arrived in a state of great agitation and told me that Lyubo Kanov had been arrested by State Security. I could hardly imagine that Lyubo would have done anything foolish in the few months since I had last seen him. Why had he been arrested? During the following days Tosho said that Lyubo's house had been searched thoroughly and a passport found. Tosho was told by his relatives that Lyubo had been arrested on charges of attempting to defect. This seemed very improbable to me but I had no reason to doubt what Tosho told me because so far everything had proved to be true. A few months ago Tosho had advised me to destroy the original copy of my short story.

Obviously that was on the advice of his relatives because Tosho knew nothing about it himself. Soon I was again summoned to the police department. Gaydarov and Uzunov interrogated me about Lyubo Kanov's attempted defection. This ridiculous show disgusted me because they knew perfectly well all that there was to know about my life and the people I met. They made no attempt to hide the fact but commented derisively about private aspects of my life. Both of them were extremely rude and Uzunov suggested sneeringly that he and Gaydarov should lock me up in a cell at the department to give me a chance to remember things better.

There was little that I could say about an attempt to defect of which I knew nothing. But under the strain of being very careful in my answers I forgot to consider the true purpose of this interrogation. There had never been any attempt to defect by Lyubo Kanov.

On 31st May 1977 after three months of detention, Lyubo Kanov was sentenced to prison for a year and a half on charges of having made *anti-Soviet statements*. Five years after leaving prison I am glad to say that Lyubo finally succeeded in defecting and emigrated to the United States where he established himself successfully as a psychiatrist.

I saw Gaydarov for the last time at Lyubo's trial. Gaydarov seemed very pleased with the results of a year's work. His comments were pithy and he informed me that the State Security had imposed a ban on me forbidding me to travel abroad for at least ten years.

After this trial which took less than an hour, I went for a long walk. Spring had arrived and the trees were green. I tried to imagine what I should do after all that had happened to me but gradually realized there was nothing. Still I knew the title of that part of my story that I would dedicate to Gaydarov. It would be *Vocation: Bastard*.

Chapter Nine
The Unattainable Calm

By the Spring of 1977 at the age of thirty-three, I finally had to admit that I had dedicated a decade of my life to trying in vain to escape from Bulgaria. After eleven failed attempts that had completely disrupted my life, there was little left of my dreams for the future.

Wondering what I should do next, I concluded that I might have to continue to live in Bulgaria for some time despite all my bitterness and revulsion. Up to that time my mind had been fully occupied in developing a plan to emigrate and I had been able to summon all my strength for this. In the future however I saw little reason to continue living in a society dominated by communist ideology.

At that time no-one even considered that communism might one day collapse. I too did not believe that I could witness such a profound change in my lifetime. I had firmly decided that I would not compromise with the communist system even if that entailed my continuing complete isolation and rejection. My choice seemed totally unreasonable but yet nothing would make me change my mind. I continued to live in the old attic where my first attempt to defect had been planned and continued to ask myself how I would survive during the indeterminate period remaining for me to spend in Bulgaria. At this time I was only able to emigrate to an imaginary world based on scraps of information from life beyond the hermetically-sealed borders of my country.

The only hope for a breakthrough was vested in possible interest in my patent abroad. Although I believed absolutely in my engine design I felt it was impossible to continue in my position as an unemployed inventor holding a private patent. A *Committee on Technical Progress* dealt with inventions and patents in Bulgaria and issued me with a permit granting me exclusive rights on the engine but refusing to lend any further support. On 25th August 1977 my patent was registered abroad and some time later I received a copy of the West German *Offenlegungschrift*, within whose orange pages it was described.

However as time went by, no interest was shown in my patented design and I came to believe that the only way to obtain a direct response from motorcar manufacturers would be by approaching them individually. At that point, another bureaucratic quagmire stretched before me; the patent had been issued personally to me yet the monopoly of the exploitation of patents was vested in a state company existing solely to trade in licences. Its officials refused to even listen to me on the basis that my patent had not been included in the current annual plan of the company. It was fairly obvious too that no-one intended to incorporate it at any time in the future either.

At last after endless negotiation another state company agreed to handle the matter. It had the pompous title of *The Progress Centre for Accelerated Implementation* that produced a hilarious abbreviation in Bulgarian. The company was intended to profit from overcoming the delays that the sluggish bureaucratic machine placed in the path of new technologies by using the personal contacts of its manager, a distinguished member of the Party *nomenclatura*.

The Progress Centre would see to it that my invention was included in their plan for promoting patents but could not take any further responsibility either by building a prototype or by meeting the cost of the registration procedure. For my part I would be required to transfer my rights in the patent to The Centre in return for which I would be entitled to twenty per cent of prospective profits and the right to approve all proposed transactions. No-one with a private patent could dream of a similar contract but naturally I would not expect to earn a penny if no buyer turned up.

I reflected on Richard III offering his kingdom for a horse after losing that last battle. My situation was no better than his for no-one seemed to care whether my invention could be profitable and most particularly no-one was interested to deal with a patent so totally opposed to the communist ideal of an invention. Nevertheless I signed a contract accepting all these conditions. In exchange I received a letter informing me that on 3rd November my invention was included in the outline plan of the *Technica Foreign Trade Society* for promoting Bulgarian patents abroad. At last at the beginning of 1978 five motor companies were approached with an offer to build a prototype of the engine with my cooperation. They were General Motors, Ford, American Motors, Fiat and Peugeot. I could see no reason why other firms should not be offered the same opportunity but at Technica no-one seemed to consider that necessary.

All I could do now was to wait patiently and because that could take years, I began work on the scale model of the prototype. Maybe it was an artistic need that persuaded me to do that. I could happily spend hours creating every single part and my efforts finally resulted in a beautiful compact model that would require very precise manufacturing technology in production.

I also resumed my work on theoretical physics. It took me some considerable time to regain the levels that I had reached in 1972. Looking back I felt a pang of regret for I had missed the chance to work on theoretical physics at the Berkeley Institute of Technology. Nevertheless since that first publication of my ideas my concepts had further evolved and I was now eager to present them in a way that would be found more accessible.

One day I began to write a short story in which my narrator gave an account of his life by discussing as he went along ideas on theoretical physics in a populist manner. The theory that fascinated him was presented in several paragraphs defined by little arrows. My narrator's story took an absurd turn when I obliged him to marry a perfect replica of my second wife. I added various explicit if not obscene details to the story which made me laugh out loud. The title of my piece was *The Unattainable Calm of a Salesman*.

I derived great pleasure in writing that bizarre story during the long days of awaiting an answer from the motor industry abroad. I had no intention to publish it and yet a blank space had been left at the point where my hero drew his conclusions about the communist system. Further on I explained to the reader that this was because of the heretical character of his conclusions. In an earlier story I had explicitly stated my own feelings about the communist system and a commentary about that story had undoubtedly been added to the files kept on me by State Security.

In fact on reflection I consider that my life was even more bizarre than the fiction of *The Unattainable Calm*.

It was my third year in the old attic with rickety furniture after my years as a student. I had a hard wooden bed taking up half the room, a small creaking table, a chair and a small cabinet. The furniture was all much older than I and at one time I had painted them brown. My pictures of prewar motor cars hanging on the walls did little to relieve the impression of over-

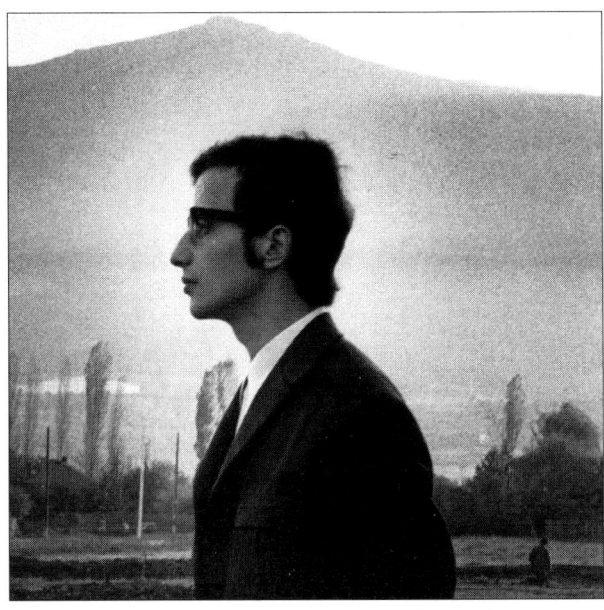

Reflecting (1970) on problems of theoretical physics

Movie art director in 1973

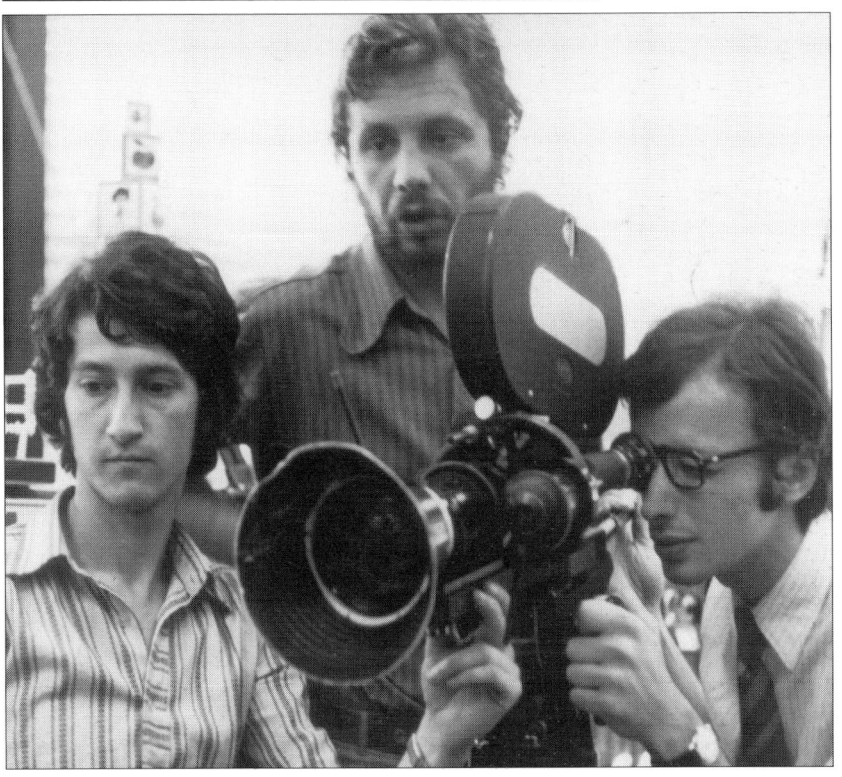

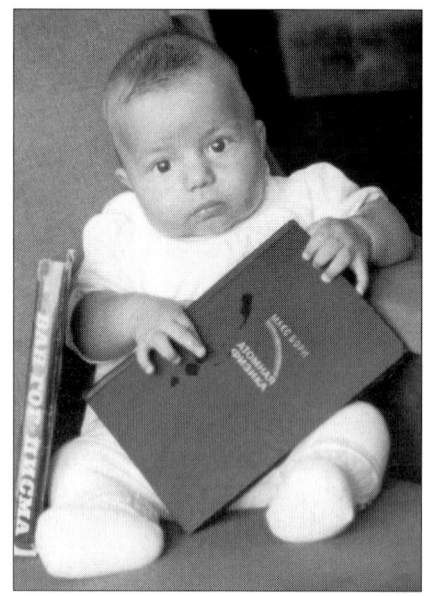

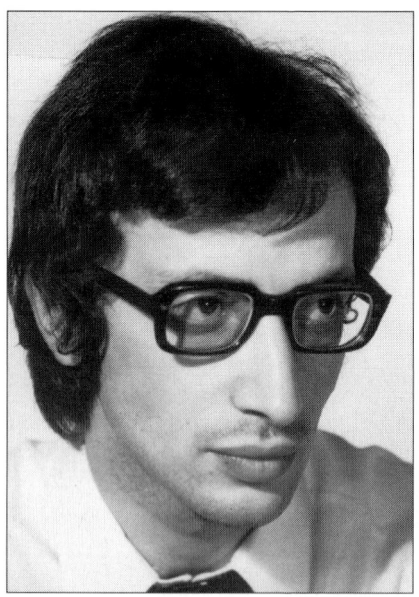

My son Viktor holding Max Born's 'Nuclear Physics' and the letters of van Gogh

Aged twenty-nine

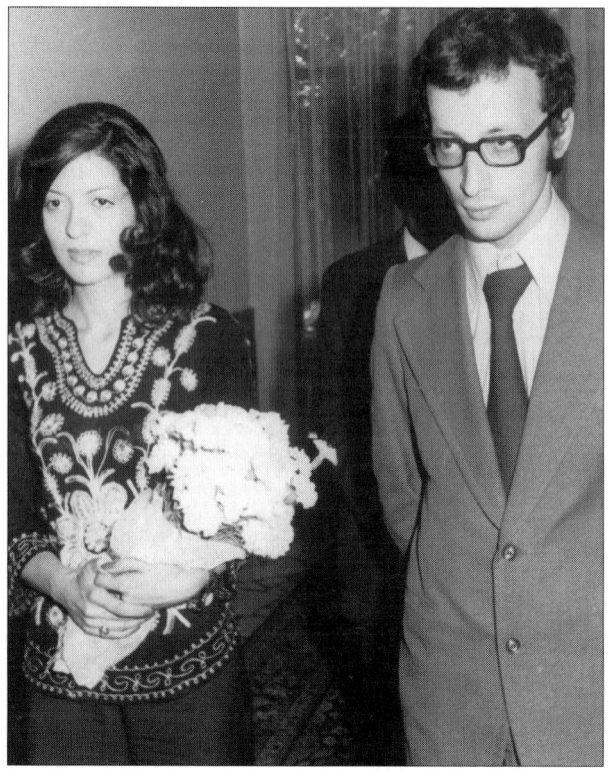

My marriage to Galya

In 1979 I began my experiments with 'M'

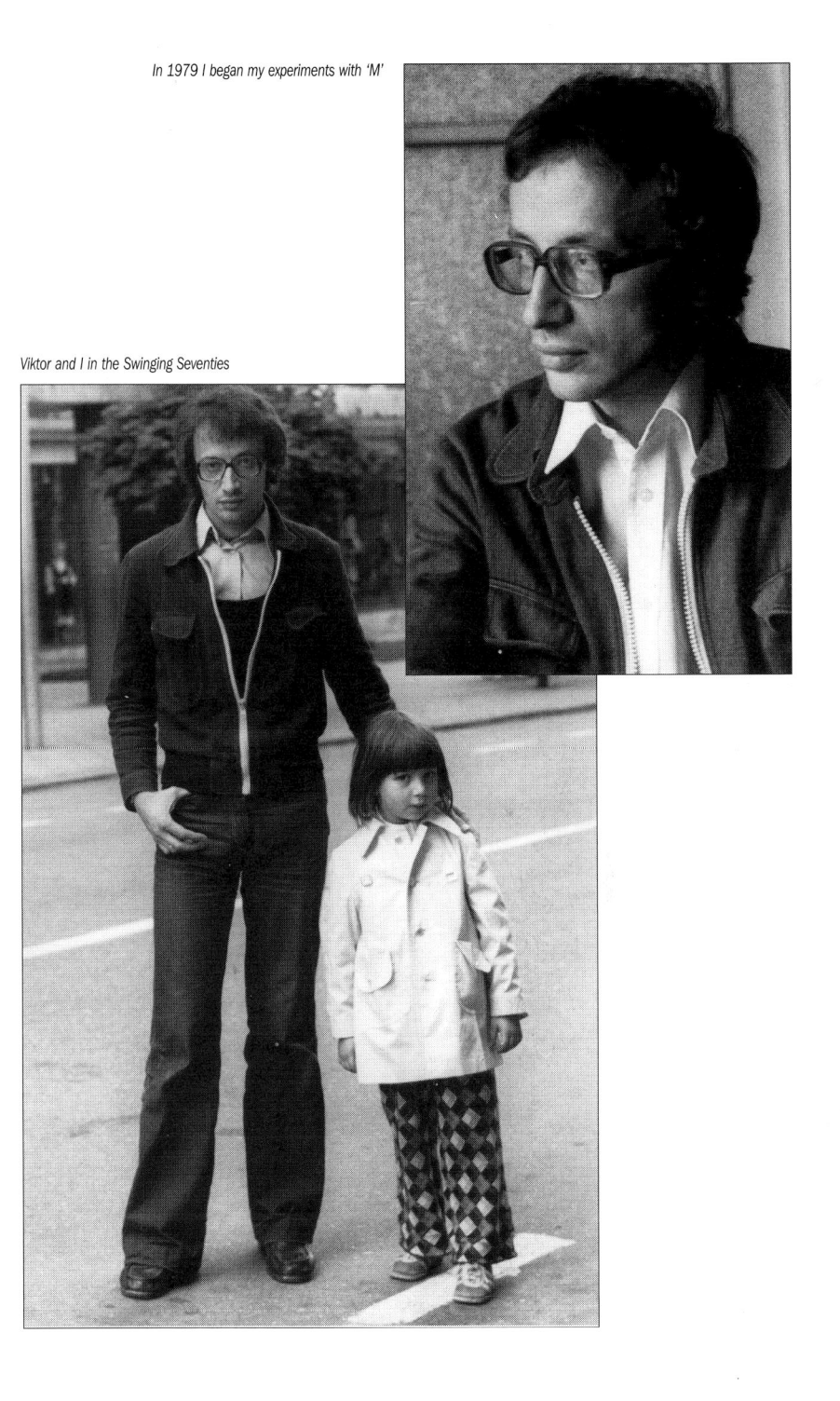

Viktor and I in the Swinging Seventies

Roxanne

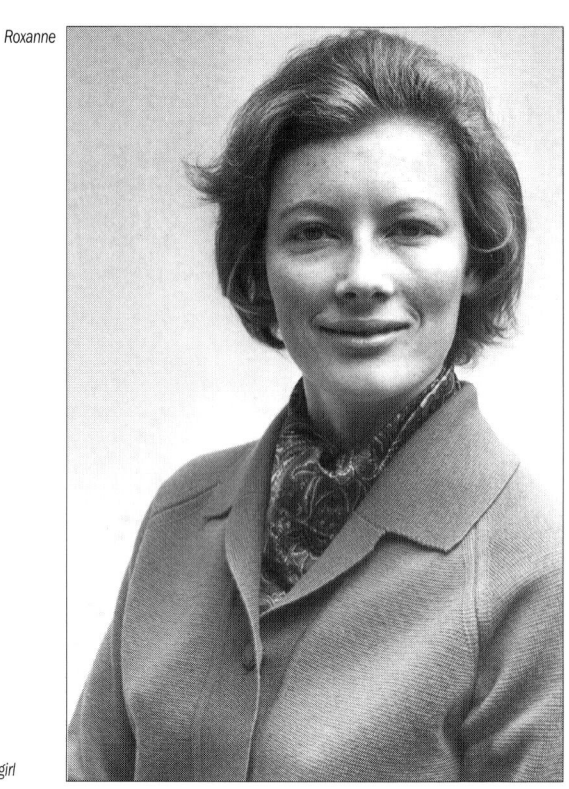

In 1986 I considered marriage to a foreign girl

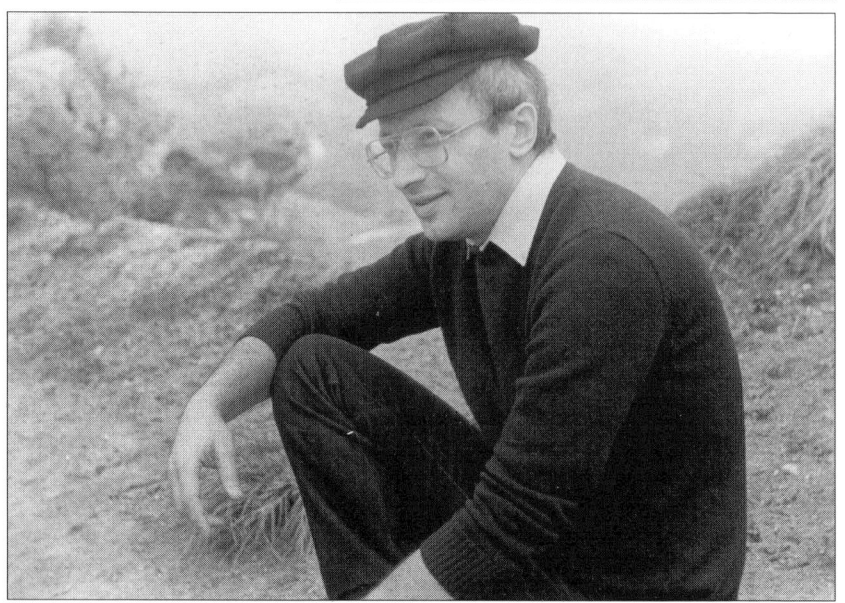

The Unattainable Calm

all shabbiness and decay created by the uneven whitewashed walls and cracked window panes. An ill-fitting hardboard door separated me from the narrow corridor outside which was even more depressing and grimy than my living quarters.

Rising above all that in the tiny space left I constructed scale models inspired by the motor cars of my childhood. Usually they were small two-door coupés like the old *Fiat Topolino* with rakish lines that recalled prewar sports cabriolets. For years on end during the late sleepless hours I would draw sketches of the same subject over and over again. It was a hobby or just simple art; a pastime without practical application but nevertheless it gave me great pleasure. The disadvantage was that the process of making these models added dust and wood chippings to the clutter of my miserable attic.

A drawing board, typewriter and a few books completed the tiny world in which I waited for the day that General Motors and Ford would respond to my licence offer and I would leave for Detroit.

It was not allowed that I should follow up the contacts made with the motor car companies. During February of 1978, Technica informed me that the offer letters had been sent by a Mr Georgiev. It was obvious to me that he disliked this job and was particularly unpleasant to me, assuring me that telephoning Technica made little sense - I must simply wait for them to call me in the event of a response.

In March General Motors, Ford and American Motors received the offer and asked Technica to sign a document containing standard conditions before taking further steps. The document was signed and returned in April. Then a letter was received from General Motors announcing that it was not interested in acquiring rights to the patent but would reconsider the offer if experimental results were available. The letter to Ford became lost in the files and a year passed before that company asked for more information about the patent. American Motors ignored the approach; Peugeot and Fiat wrote to announce that they had no interest in it. However, no-one took the trouble to inform me personally although I telephoned Technica regularly and asked for information.

Peugeot and Fiat having turned down the offer and only General Motors showing the slightest interest, in November 1978 the Committee for Technical Progress decided that it was time to bring the matter to an end. The registration procedure was suspended on the pretext that I had failed to pay the expenses in hard currency. Besides this Committee decided to start a legal action against me for failing to meet my obligations but naturally no-one bothered to inform me of those decisions either.

It was clear to me that the bureaucratic machine had decided to keep me in the dark as part of its strategy. The year drew to an end and every time that I called Technica I was told that there was still no answer to their offer and I patiently waited for another month before calling again. This hide-and-seek process continued into the following year and it was not until March 1979 that I was finally told the truth. There was very little for me to be enthusiastic about.

As I stared through the attic window at the pouring spring rain I asked myself whether this was the end of the road for me as an inventor; a road on which I had set out twenty years ago when I heard the news about Wankel's engine on a jammed broadcast from a foreign radio station. Obviously I had lost the battle and would not be given another chance by the authorities. But I refused to come to terms with that thought and continued for a long time to study the roofs and peeling windowless walls of the houses opposite my attic. In the end I decided that I would not give up despite not having the faintest idea of how to proceed. I sat at my typewriter, took a piece of paper and began a letter to the Committee for Technical Progress.

The first thing I had to do was to save the registration procedure. I had agreed to pay for it in hard currency purely because I had no other choice. But where could I obtain foreign currency if I were not allowed to leave the country? At the time foreign currency could only be purchased on the black market and that was illegal. This seemed to provide me with an argument: as long as I was prevented from going abroad no one could withhold my rights to the patent simply because I had no foreign currency to pay for registration. The decision to suspend the procedure abroad was therefore unlawful and I insisted on renewing it, pointing out that I could only pay for it in Bulgarian levs.

More than a year previously I had signed a contract transferring my rights in the patent to two state organisations, The Centre and Technica, in exchange for their commitment to secure the widest possible exploitation of my invention. By reluctantly sending letters to only five companies they had in my view neglected their obligation. Besides this, neither of them had signed the contract. I had not heard a thing from The Centre and the events of the previous year demonstrated that the contract had not been taken seriously and neither had my patent rights and my invention. Because the contract had simply been ignored I felt it was my right to declare it invalid.

I sent off a letter with those arguments insisting that the registration procedure be renewed. I pressed the Committee for Technical Progress to comply with the law and pointed out that it was liable for all consequential damages. I knew that my letter would hardly cause concern at the Committee. Its chairman Nacho Papazov, a party *apparatchik,* was said to spend most of his time playing with toy trains on the scale model of the Sofia metro system that would never be built.

On 29th April I applied for a passport, explaining that I could save my rights to the invention and perhaps realize its application only by travelling to the West. I offered all future revenues to the Bulgarian state. Two weeks later I was refused a passport. Once again I applied to see the head of the passport department and was received by a colonel who explained that he personally did not mind allowing me to go abroad but the city police department had refused to countersign my application.

I was not surprised that my twelfth attempt to leave Bulgaria had failed, too. I could hardly expect State Security to have forgotten me since Inspector Lyubomir Kotsef who had led the investigation on Lyubo Kanov in the previous year was on record as having described me as `a prominent Sofia dissident'. Without a doubt, Colonel Christozko Uzunov of the Lenin district police department was well-informed of the conflict arising from my patent. I was unaware of what was in the file kept on me but the registration procedure was now surrounded by an information vacuum. For months I had received nothing from the patent lawyers abroad. The Committee for Technical Progress was also silent although I had paid the expenses of their procedure. Had the procedure been renewed or was it suspended?

To pay the expenses of the procedure in Bulgarian levs, a sum that even at the artificial rate of exchange for the US dollar in Bulgaria amounted to a five-year salary, I had traded my invention for the third time after the previous aborted deals with Nikolay and the Centre for Accelerated Implementation.

Simultaneously another Bulgarian, Stoyan Cholakov, had begun a private procedure to protect his rights in a patent. Cholakov came from the Macedonian region of South West Bulgaria. Like most inventors, he refused to give up and was quite out of touch with reality although very business-like. Cholakov had filed for a patent on an electric hoist while working for a Bulgarian state enterprise in an African country where salaries were higher and payable in foreign currency. The procedure had not only cost him his entire savings but the secret service officials

The Unattainable Calm

had quickly sent him back home to Bulgaria. Still Cholakov had hired a lawyer to protect his interests abroad. He visited me a couple of times and was considerably interested in my invention. Finally I signed a contract giving Cholakov ten per cent of my revenues while he undertook to pay for the expenses of the procedure that I had so far carried out. A contract of that kind must have been a curiosity at that time and Cholakov was probably the first Bulgarian to invest in an invention in a private capacity.

Meanwhile a director from the studios of popular scientific films came to see me to announce that he intended to make a film about my invention. I could not see any harm in that and agreed to cooperate. I even made a plexiglass scale model of the engine that could be turned by hand. The film was shot and edited in a manner which gave the impression that this was an absurd invention made even more ridiculous by an ironic comment at the end.

As the end of summer drew near I wondered whether there was anything I could do before accepting that my invented engine was doomed to failure. One last opportunity was to demonstrate the engine in person to motor companies that we had not yet approached.

I decided to present my engine to some of the Western car companies participating in the annual international fair in September at Plovdiv. Cholakov agreed enthusiastically to assist me and we left for Plovdiv taking the publication of the patent and the plexiglass scale model that I had made for the film. At the fair I succeeded in approaching the representatives of Mercedes and Volvo.

Lothar Rubenbauer was politely sceptical while I demonstrated the working of the engine on a small table on the Mercedes-Benz stand. He listened to my presentation and without further comment advised me to send information about my invention to the Mercedes patent department in Stuttgart.

Volvo was represented by a young Bulgarian whose cooperation with the secret service was obligatory and moreover could be read in his face. He was confused and continually asked me from which Bulgarian enterprise I came, as I demonstrated my engine to the Swedish engineer on the stand. The latter, whose name I can no longer remember, examined the plexiglass scale model thoroughly and seemed quite impressed. He made a copy of the document and promised to hand it to his company. I left Volvo's stand with the feeling that I had done a good job.

In November I sent letters to other motor car companies although I was not sure that my letters ever arrived. I certainly never received an answer from any of them.

My engine was also demonstrated to BMW in a rather mysterious way through Tosho's brother the truck driver. Tosho kept in touch with me but I felt that he was more circumspect than before whenever the secret service was mentioned. Once he told me that his brother knew a designer working for BMW but it was not before September that year that Tosho gave the scale model of the engine and a copy of the publication to his brother asking him to take them to that same designer in Munich. I wondered whether Tosho's relatives in the secret service had given their approval. Perhaps someone was eager to see whether I could get anywhere by personally undertaking the promotion of my engine.

In the autumn of 1979 I realised that I had done all possible to promote my design. If no one had shown any interest I must simply accept that this was the end of my four-stroke internal combustion engine invented four years before. Although I believed completely in the merit of my invention it had proved impossible to make a living as a professional inventor in Bulgaria. So far grandmother had fulfilled the role of patroness and had covered most of my daily expenses. Sometimes I had received an odd commission as an artist and everything I earned from that was ploughed back into the invention.

During those months I frequently met Shego and we would spend a couple of hours at the Shapkite café round the corner. He continued to write poetry for amusement well into his tenth year of marriage. He worked at a telephone exchange and earned extra money by taking in typing. He led a thrifty simple existence with his wife in the same flat on the third floor where once his grandparents had lived. Despite their peaceful cohabitation as husband and wife he was now madly in love with a student girl. Shego did not have the strength of purpose to abandon either of them. One day he bought a light green Skoda and would often invite me to accompany him and his girlfriend on excursions.

Bobby would often join me and Shego, too. After some years of a relatively calm existence with his wife Shego became involved in a turbulent affair with a colleague which had almost ruined his marriage for the second time. After many vicissitudes he returned to his wife in the hope that he would fall in love again with some other girl in the future. Bobby had a taste for restaurants, fine wines and expensive cigarettes. He did not mind getting into debt and was a lavish spender. He took on a job at a computing centre, showed aptitude for programming and was quickly promoted to an administrative post. The centre sent him abroad on business trips but Bobby showed no interest in defecting. He rather liked his job in fact and even managed to persuade Shego to join him at the centre.

As so many years earlier, Bobby, Shego and I now had fun recreating our humorous mythology. Everything in this fantasy world took on monstrously hilarious dimensions until we arrived at absurdities that could not be translated into plain Bulgarian. I would invent stories about Shego's life; his prolific output of verse, his amorous escapades and his plodding relationship with his dull wife. All the extravagant details that I invented had nothing to do with Shego's real life. After completing *The Unattainable Calm* I began to write stories about Shego and his fanciful adventures; they were so entertaining that they often made me roar with laughter. Shego laughed too and his kind sympathetic nature was a great comfort to me although he hardly realized that.

While joking about Shego I continued to want to find a girlfriend for myself. I had a couple of short-lived affairs with student girls that ended in failure and made me feel wretched. One day I met Tsvete, a slender shy blonde girl with blue eyes. She was a student at the Institute of Forestry and had never even dreamed of emigrating. I could not imagine that we might have a future together but our temporary relationship became more serious than each of us cared to admit. Tsvete could not always understand why I enjoyed the stories about Shego so much but she was patient with me as I wrote them.

In fact my life in general was not easy. My son was at school, his grandfather who had so far taken care of him, died. I often took Viktor to my parents and was upset by the thought that I was unable to offer him a more comfortable existence. After several years of tempestuous life with my brother's family, grandmother moved back into my parents' flat. She suffered from severe attacks of rheumatism and became increasingly immobile. Ten years after his cancer operation my father was now a very sick man while mother tried to help everyone and never ceased to worry about me.

At the end of the year Tosho said BMW had responded positively to my offer. I had known Tosho for three years but it took me a long time to get much information out of him. After several days of talking on long walks I reached the following conclusions:

The plexiglass model and the copy of the publication that Tosho was supposed to send to BMW had evidently been intercepted and thoroughly examined by the secret service, most probably with the connivance of his relatives. Tosho could tell me very little about who it was that had demonstrated my engine to BMW but having briefly met Tosho's brother a year earlier I could hardly imagine him doing that.

The Unattainable Calm

I concluded that BMW had sent a letter responding positively to my engine. The Secret Service had most probably obtained the letter and the chances were that I would never see it. Tosho had probably been instructed to say exactly what he had already told me and that was probably all he knew.

Something strange was happening to the response of another company too. I contacted the representatives of Mercedes and Volvo to ask about any news on my offer. Mercedes politely turned it down but I found the letter in my postbox only a week later. Volvo however did not reply. The young representative whom I had met at the Plovdiv fair said that I would soon receive an answer but when I went to see him in his office at the end of the year he was very excited and two of his bosses came to shake me by the hand. After I left the office I received a small model Volvo car that Santa Claus had sent as a present for my son; I never received a letter from Volvo. It seemed hardly possible to me that the Swedish engineer would not reply after he had taken my letter and a copy of the publication of my patent. A negative answer would most certainly find its way to my postbox. What had happened to Volvo's letter? Tosho knew nothing.

At the end of 1979 I reached the conclusion that I must have succeeded in attracting the attention of a car company by just sending a drawing and a description covering ten pages. It seemed almost improbable, however. I drank a bottle of brandy with Bobby and Shego but all I could do was wait to see what might happen.

In the first days of the new year, Bulgarian television broadcast the film about my invention. There must have been something going on with my design while I was being kept in the dark. I did not like this at all. A former classmate whom I had not seen for nearly twenty years seemed very eager to help me build a prototype of the engine. He worked at a glassworks and in his free time built small two-stroke engines for the National Aero-Modelling team. He suggested that he could build a small working prototype of my engine. At our second meeting he was accompanied by an army colonel who openly offered me the opportunity to work for a top-secret research institute. A rumour then reached Bobby that our former classmate had boasted to a girlfriend that he was an officer in the Secret Service and had shown her his gun. After meeting him a couple of times I decided he might very well have told the truth. He suggested that I send a request to President Zhivkov through an acquaintance of his pointing out that the Party leader was the only person who could now help me.

I had no doubt that it was probable that Zhivkov was the only person who could help me but I seriously doubted that he would have any sympathy for my type. All I could do was to wait to see what the secret service had in store for me. I did not have to wait long for soon Tosho told me that Colonel Uzunov wanted to see me. I did not feel like meeting him again but Tosho warned me that if I refused I might instead be arrested.

So once again I found myself in the office of Colonel Uzunov where three years ago the attempt had been made to steal my rights to the invention. This time the meeting was attended by an army colonel whom I had not met before. He discussed at length my dazzling prospects if I would agree to work for a top-secret research institute. Was this not the same institute of which I had already heard? BMW was not mentioned but the new model of the Soviet *Zaporozhets* car was highly praised. At the end of the meeting he insisted that I should accept his offer to join the research institute.

All this reminded me of Kafka's *The Trial*.

When I analysed the situation I reached several conclusions. In 1976 my invention had aroused the interest of the secret service and certain ambitious lackeys like Gaydarov had seized it as an opportunity to advance their own career. Later, possibly under the influence of the secret service, Technica was willing to promote the invention abroad to see whether it might produce results. However the bureaucratic machine simply sought a way to rid itself of the entire affair and brought the matter to a conclusion by rejecting any potential advantages the engine might have. As the car industry abroad seemed to show interest in it, the secret service could argue that it should take the matter into its own hands. It had decided to send me to work for a secret institute so that it could seize my patent rights. It mattered not whether I liked the idea; I would simply be forced to accept the offer and State Security would see to that.

At that time the State Security organization would use threats and compromising material to blackmail people into cooperating. A police investigation would be threatened if they refused to act as informers. Prison sentences could be reduced, careers made and privileges granted in exchange for cooperation. Human lives could be disrupted by blackmail; there were reported cases of suicide too. Many people were unable to resist the pressure and agreed to carry the burden of spying, blackmailing and morally tormenting their fellow citizens. This was the fate of hundreds of thousands of Bulgarians who were not professed communists. Still there were always people who would volunteer to cooperate.

The blackmail specialists were now busy persuading me to work for the top-secret research institute. Colonel Uzunov, with responsibility for me, had developed his career using Lenin's method of terror and violence on stubborn unyielding people to forcing them to accept communist ideas. He was probably very good at this. With his experience, he now prepared for me a nightmare with more hardships than anything I had seen so far and all that because foreign companies seemed to have shown an interest in my invention.

I was now thirty-six and knew that I would not give in to the pressure despite the price that I would have to pay for resistance.

Above all, these developments meant that my invention was doomed never to see daylight. In the name of *the ideological struggle* I was not to be allowed to work with Western companies and my engine had no chance of ever being built and tried. The letters that never reached me were filed in the archives of the secret service along with the other files on millions of Bulgarians. To this very day these files have not been opened to the public. As I write these lines twenty years later I can still not add anything to my speculation at the time nor can I answer the questions that haunted me. In the hands of the secret service my patent was doomed to oblivion by my refusal to work for the secret research institute.

On the other hand, I would now most certainly be further intimidated and repressed before the State Security finally realized that I would not give in. Tosho frankly admitted to me that the people who had decided to blackmail me were very cruel and determined to use all possible means at their disposal including sending me to prison where I would be forced to continue to work on the drawings of my engine in return for an occasional bowl of beans. That meant that I would be further isolated and my friends intimidated, like Lyubo Kanov. I had already received threats that my sister whom I loved dearly might be in trouble because of my behaviour. There was no doubt that I was now in a very difficult position. It seemed that the time spent writing *The Unattainable Calm* had probably been the best period in my life during recent years.

The spring of 1980 came and Tosho asked me regularly whether I would agree to see Colonel Uzunov once again. In the end State Security accepted that my refusal was final and decided to take the next step. I was summoned to the Lenin District Police Department on 2nd April; the next round in the struggle had begun.

While awaiting the confrontation I worked furiously during every day, hour and minute left to me. I was in a hurry to complete the text of a discovery I had recently made entitled *A Micro-organism causing Atherosclerosis and many other ailments*.

Chapter Ten
Candida Albicans

Consideration of the structure of the human body has aroused controversy throughout history. Even today, although so many of their secrets have been revealed, we are not completely sure how human genes work. As far as biological theory is concerned it lags far behind other areas; most hypotheses in biology resemble suppositions by comparison with the precise and well-structured theories of physics. Whilst the theory of classical mechanics came into being three hundred years ago, only in the last century Louis Pasteur and Robert Koch were ridiculed by colleagues for their claim to have discovered bacteria and their role in infectious diseases. At that time all the great names in medicine firmly believed that microorganisms developed spontaneously in the diseased body.

Throughout the twentieth century medicine has waged war against the microorganisms responsible for a wide range of diseases. Attacked by sulphonamides and antibiotics, bacteria however tend to adapt to every new generation of drugs and remain a serious threat to human health. Viruses whose role among living organisms is not yet fully understood, can cause dangerous epidemics. In the world of microorganisms inhabiting the human body there is also a role for all forms of fungi and yeasts; none of which has ever been considered seriously harmful to human health.

As fungi differ greatly from all other organisms it is difficult to position them in the tree of evolution. Generally speaking they resemble plants although lacking chlorophyll and feeding on substances extracted from other organisms. Today medicine believes that although fungi are widely present in the human body they only cause disorders in certain cases. It is not yet clear why in some cases fungi remain dormant while in others they cause infection or mycoses, although immune deficiency and reduced resistance after treatment by drugs are seen as important contributing factors. Most mycoses are considered harmless although they are persistent and strongly resistant to treatment.

During recent years mycoses have increasingly appeared during pregnancy and childbirth; affecting both mother and child. The fungus causing mycosis in newborn babies was discovered by Robin in the mid-nineteenth century and was named *Odium albicans* by him. However in 1939 the name of the fungus was changed to *Candida albicans*; more generally known as *white fungus*. Since its discovery it has been generally accepted that *Candida albicans* does not cause problems in the human body except in certain cases of heavy mycosis. Antibiotics reducing natural human resistance have encouraged the increase in *Candida* cases in recent times. This fungus is not however a `hot topic' in medicine. However at the end of 1979 I was faced with many questions deriving from it.

Ever since childhood I have suffered from chronic sinusitis that intensified each winter. I was routinely treated with various antibiotics that often had strong and unpleasant side effects, particularly affecting my stomach and intestinal tract. In 1979 after several extended antibiotic treatment regimes I was found to have developed a mycosis. I began taking a maximum dose of 'M', an anti-fungal antibiotic *(see warning after title page)*.

During the first week of treatment my condition immediately improved. 'M' was prescribed for up to two weeks and I was authorised to repeat the treatment. I continued to take the drug as long as I felt an improvement.

By the end of the third week a thick layer of dead epithelial cells began to peel from my face and the palms of my hands when I took a bath. One day while vigorously rubbing the skin of my face to remove the peeling layer, I discerned a strange pattern appearing on my skin - two small wounds received at the time that my jaw had been broken became visible, eighteen years after the event.

What was happening? I observed that generally 'M' caused intensive shedding of dead epithelial cells from my skin. The small wounds on my face were in fact purple-tinted patches of dead tissue that easily peeled from my skin. I was certain that the dead tissue did not result from the influence of 'M' but most probably had been there hidden within my skin in some way for many years. When I inspected the strange pale purple stains on my face I began to realise that this was a mysterious phenomenon. Whatever it was that was happening to me could not be explained by current understanding of fungi or the accepted effects of 'M'. I therefore developed a hypothesis that could explain the phenomenon.

The fungus that I had treated with 'M' probably connected dead cells to my tissue by its very existence. 'M' counteracted the fungoid activity and my body then rejected the dead cells. I could find no similar hypothesis in accepted medicine so I determined to put it to the test. For the time being it was sufficient to continue taking 'M' and observing the effect. It was now early 1980.

As a result of my continuing experiment my face soon looked dreadful. Small sores with hard red and purple crusts covered my entire left cheek, nose and forehead. These were the places where I had been wounded. Each day crusts peeled away revealing new yet larger ones that would peel off during the following day. The process continued for weeks and the very sight of it was terrifying. Nevertheless it provided me with the evidence I needed to support my hypothesis. These crusts were deposits of strangely coloured dead tissue released by my skin. Finally after a few weeks a normal layer of skin appeared and the sores vanished without scars.

I began a second month of experiment. The phenomenon I had witnessed resembled nothing I had ever seen or read about. I was convinced that the process of rejecting dead tissue and generating new normal tissue in replacement was linked entirely to the taking of 'M' and influenced by the amount of the daily dose. What was happening to my face was clearly related to those old physical wounds; it was not my skin that changed. Breaking my jaw obviously had profound consequences and the dead tissue peeling off could hardly have had a beneficial effect on my health while it remained. At that point I considered another question: how did the medical profession consider dead tissue?

In asking myself that question I suddenly appreciated that I could be on the brink of a fundamental discovery.

Dead tissue is found throughout the human body; in the skin, the mucous membrane, and the internal organs. Similar dead, hardened tissue forms *atheromatous plaques* inside the blood vessels which are the most frequent cause of death in developed countries. Today the medical profession does not consider that dead tissue throughout the human body has a common link; dead tissue is considered to be the consequence of a range of diseases. Atheromatous plaques are not even regarded as a disease but rather as the manifestation of sclerosis, the seemingly natural process of the constant accumulation of dead tissue in the ageing human body. The reasons for premature sclerosis in the blood vessels remain largely unknown although stress, smoking and certain types of diet are considered to increase the risk of its development.

I therefore asked myself whether all these accumulations of dead tissue in the human body could be caused simply by fungoid activity.

Late one evening I was examining some of the hard crusts detaching from the sores on my face and wondered whether they had anything in common with the hard plaques blocking the aorta which frequently cause heart attacks.

I decided that they were very probably one and the same.

After thinking carefully, I came to the conclusion that if my hypothesis could indeed be proved right the world was an absurd place. I began the task of testing my hypothesis.

I obtained from a postmortem section a piece of human tissue containing atheromatous plaques. In one of these plaques I made a small incision and treated it with *Canesten*, a liquid anti-fungal drug. The plaque proceeded to swell and the hardened tissue began to disintegrate - something that even powerful solvents had failed to achieve.

This indeed was evidence supporting my hypothesis.

I continued to take 'M' and noticed a series of visible deteriorations or curative crises occurring in old wounds probably because of the peeling away of dead tissue. My sinusitis that was revealed in an X-ray photograph as dark spots then deteriorated and the secretion intensified. A similar process was taking place in my throat. Old wounds on my legs shed dead cells too. Obviously there was a general process of dead tissue rejection taking place throughout my body. What was going on in my blood vessels? Were they becoming clogged by loose tissue? My skin and surface blood vessels changed colour at 24 hour intervals and I often felt dizzy and sleepy.

On examining decomposing dead tissue I discerned filaments clearly visible to the naked eye. These threads resembled extraordinarily large formations of the fungus. I kept some of them for future use. The fungus formed structures that seemed to be larger and more fully developed than those so far described in the literature and this brought me to the idea that dead tissue was probably contained by the fungus providing it with a hiding place - these large thread-like structures could only be seen if the dead tissue itself decomposed. I imagined that the fungus united the dead cells to form an environment in which it could feed and reproduce while remaining attached to the human tissue. In the last century Vihrov described filiform structures in sclerotic dead tissue, but so far no-one had suggested that those structures could be fungal.

My experiment continued into a third month. Thus far I had observed various stages of the process and could compare this evidence with my theory. It appeared that various forms of dead tissue were connected in a complex system throughout the body and represented more than just a layer which peeled off simultaneously. It seemed that there were numerous accumulations of dead tissue throughout the entire body at varying depths with particular concentrations in the area of old wounds and sores. They were slowly rejected over and over again at precisely the same points. I realised that this process could perhaps continue for many years.

At that stage in my experimentation I assumed that the fungus active within the body was not considered as a disease in the sense of the current medical definition of human disorders. It was possible that having gained access to the embryo in the mother's womb the fungus continued as a parasite in all humans. Many of the processes that could be observed in the normal ageing of the human body such as a general accumulation of dead tissue and sclerosis were most probably the results of this continuous parasitic symbiosis. Was it possible that the fungus had travelled with man throughout his evolution? Was it possible indeed that it affected other biological species too? These questions intrigued me but went too far - for the time being my hypothesis was restricted to the possibility that the fungus occurred parasitically in human beings from birth. In such a case the current definition of health implied that the parasitic symbiosis of the fungus within the human body was in a state of equilibrium. Any disruption resulting from increased generation of dead tissue in certain areas was probably a by-product of diseases. For example, the fact that heart disease is the most common cause of death in developed countries lent support to my hypothesis. Heart attacks and strokes increase with the growing use of antibiotics which indirectly stimulate the fungus, probably leading to disturbance of the balance in the human body.

I decided to seek volunteers to assist me. I explained my theory to two young men and they agreed to carry out my experiment using smaller doses of 'M'. One had had a serious burn on his left arm and I was able to observe that all that happened to my face occurred around the area of his old wound. All other effects were repeated down to the smallest detail. Then I began to experiment with my son Viktor who also suffered from severe sinusitis which had to that point resisted treatment with antibiotics.

By the end of the third month of experiment I reached the conclusion that I had sufficient evidence at my disposal to support my theory. There remained the question of what to do with it. It was now mid-March 1980 and I was summoned to report at the Lenin Police Department in two weeks where I knew that I would be forced to work for a leading secret research institute.

One cold morning I sat at the deserted *Shapkite* café smoking a cigarette and drinking a cup of lukewarm coffee while I pondered what to do next. I had never imagined that my life could take such a strange turn. I felt that I would be unable to deal with the ordeal awaiting me. Despite my scientific interests, I felt that what I really wanted to do was to spend the summer with a pretty girl at the seaside. Instead I was now involved in a new experiment and a new theory in medicine compared with which my work on theoretical physics and the design of four-stroke engines seemed like a harmless pastime. My theory could be simply tested in any laboratory but fundamental changes in modern medical practice were not easy to achieve. At the time I could not imagine being able to convince any responsible authority in Sofia that as a result of solitary research in an attic I had arrived at a revolutionary discovery; the cause of many diseases and an effective drug to treat them. It appeared to me that there was only one place where I could be taken seriously - by the secret service. That powerful body could test my theory immediately and my work in pursuit of this theory might possibly be the only argument which would allow me to avoid joining the secret research institute. Would the secret service help me to advance my theory? Its interference might be dangerous but it was not going to leave me alone in any case. Having analysed the position, I realised that there was only one thing for me to do.

I downed my now cold coffee and telephoned Tosho. Without a word he carried my message to the secret service: I was eager to demonstrate to them a discovery in medicine. I sat at the typewriter and elaborated my hypothesis and experiments in a thirty page memorandum.

A few days later a State Security officer whom I had not previously met came to see me. I was given to understand that this Slavcho Protogerov had taken over my heavy file from

Gaydarov. Protogerov was a pleasant young man; a former professional soccer player with a constant smile and a calm, relaxed nature. He talked little and noted down my theory which I explained to him when we met in the City Garden. Finally, I gave him my memorandum and he took it, still marked with corrections, and continued on his secret way.

A long period of silence followed. Tosho had no news for me.

On 2 April I was summoned to report at the Lenin District Police Department. Colonel Uzunov awaited me in his office. The moment I saw him I knew we would not be discussing the secret research institute or my four-stroke engine. If I was not mistaken, my research into the fungus had altered the Colonel's outlook beyond recognition. He repeated constantly that he could not understand how the great science of medicine had failed to discover such a simple fact. Uzunov lacked the knowledge to judge my experiment but he undoubtedly firmly believed in my theory. Despite his sly, hypocritical manner, there was a certain benevolence in his words. However the greatest surprise came as our meeting drew to a close. Uzunov told me that his daughter suffered from severe asthma. A couple of times she had been on the verge of suffocation and doctors had advised an operation. Uzunov became visibly excited and confused while explaining this to me and begged me to go to see his daughter at home. The Colonel had begun to give her two tablets of 'M' every morning. I had not expected events would take such a turn.

Without question the article that I had given to Protogerov had been examined by medical specialists and had caused a major upheaval once it had been checked. I had taken a dazzling step forward in my non-existent career as a scientist in the eyes of the secret service. Uzunov had lost his composure; instead of blackmailing me into working for the secret institute he had now actually asked me to treat his daughter. Although my theory had not yet been openly confirmed, at least for the moment the pressure to join the research institute had evaporated. What else might I expect?

That evening immediately after my visit to the Lenin District Police Department I went to Colonel Uzunov's home. His daughter, a twenty year-old student, did indeed suffer from a serious form of asthma. I expected that treatment with 'M' would result in more serious bouts before she felt any improvement. The treatment could continue for months and severe complications or even asphyxiation could not be excluded. It was beyond my power to help if anything went wrong. I was forced to explain to Uzunov that I could not guarantee any improvement in her condition but he persisted in demanding that I carry out theexperiment on his daughter. She had tried all cures offered by the medical profession but with no benefit. I was now invited to act as daily medical consultant. The situation allowed me little room for manoeuvre, so I agreed.

I began to visit Uzunov's home each day as I waited for his daughter's first curative crisis as well as the anticipated move from the secret service. Uzunov was still highly secretive in manner and vaguely promised that I would soon be given the chance to conduct experiments to prove my theory. I was still working on a more detailed paper describing my theory and experiments which I intended to send to the Bulgarian Academy of Science. I hoped that I could find a physician or biologist who could corroborate my pathological experiment on decomposing atheromatous plaques and other specimens of dead tissue. It was easy to carry out biological experiments to identify the fungus and so far I had done this by causing the decomposition of dead tissue. The fungus could also be identified by cultivating sterile tissue from cadavers in a suitable nutrient. I felt certain that the secret service had already carried out similar experiments on their own account.

One afternoon Uzunov asked me to carry out an experiment on his daughter's sputum. An unmarked Lada police car took me to Dianabad, a sports compound with swimming pool in a housing estate on the outskirts of Sofia where it transpired there was a medical laboratory on the premises. A few men in white coats awaited us but did not introduce themselves. One asked what I required for the experiment and I asked for liquid Canesten and a glass dish. I then treated the sputum with the drug. One of the white-coated men offered me a microscope and it took me some time to adjust this professional equipment since most of my research so far had been carried out with a small low-powered school microscope. The men stood by watching me silently. Finally I located a thread of the fungus and a piece of a Y-formation specific to it. I asked the men to look through the microscope but none uttered a single word. The driver returned me to the city centre.

It appeared that this mysterious experiment was intended to put me to the test. Uzunov did not refer to it again and carefully avoided discussing any other experiments that might support my theory. I continued to visit his daughter daily and judging by the colour of her skin I assumed that the 'M' was taking its full effect. A curative crisis might occur at any moment. Then at II o'clock one evening Uzunov telephoned and asked me to come immediately. I found his daughter in the grip of a terrible asthmatic attack. I was unable to help her in any way but my presence seemed to calm her and gradually after midnight her cough subsided. Uzunov was visibly affected and promised me with tears in his eyes that if her condition improved he would personally take me to President Zhivkov and do anything I asked. He obviously loved his daughter greatly. As I left early in the morning I felt that his daughter would probably suffer further attacks and it was difficult to say how long that process might continue. After all I was still into the fourth month of experimenting on myself and still suffered recurring pain at all points where once I had wounds and still the sores on my face continued to peel off dead tissue. The other volunteers and my son taking part in the experiment also found that the process moved extremely slowly.

On the following morning I again met Uzunov in his office at the Police Department. I insisted that we discuss how I should continue my research and experiments including that on his daughter. In the beginning Uzunov had promised to help me obtain the support of medical specialists who would verify my experiments using decomposing dead tissue in a laboratory. It would only take a day to carry out these experiments but so far no attempt had been made to do so. I then told him that I thought it dangerous to continue my experiments on volunteers in uncontrolled conditions. I pointed out that I wanted to publish my theory and the experiment as soon as possible and asked him whether he himself or the secret service could help me.

Uzunov looked impassively out of his window and remarked that it would be interesting to know how medical experts would regard my work. He grinned inanely just as he had done after Lyubo Kanov's investigation. Uzunov reminded me of an impertinent, cunning peasant with no interest in promises and honour. He was in charge of my file; perhaps he was the man who had decided my destiny ever since the original State Security investigation of 1961. What might I expect from him or his superiors? I had no answer to that question and if there was any research being carried out on my theory I was kept in the dark about it. The secret service appeared to support my work and may even have sought a way to publicize it. If it did it seemed in no hurry but at least did nothing against me. Maybe men higher up in the organisation who had protected me years ago had gained more influence and power. Might it be that a kind-hearted Protogerov had infiltrated the ambitious Gaydarov into my life in an attempt to avoid conflict because of my views?

Uzunov said nothing, however. On the following day he asked me to provide a summary of my theory with suggestions for a research programme and how it should be conducted. In response I wrote to say that discoveries of this importance were not made every day and that the health of millions of people could depend on early publication although the treatment itself could only be applied after many years of research. Visibly pained, Uzunov informed me that his department was quite capable of deciding what to do. Nevertheless he accepted my article and I continued my daily visits to his daughter.

Still nothing happened. It was obvious that I could no longer rely on vague promises. Although I would have preferred to have carried out more work to obtain evidence in support, I sent on 23 May a description of my theory and experiments to the Bulgarian Academy of Science. On 27 May I received a letter from them directing me to the Medical Academy which was the authority on such matters, and to which I therefore wrote three days later.

At the same time I attempted to contact a medical specialist who could certify my experiments on atheromatous plaques. I knew a pathologist who certainly did not share my enthusiasm for my discovery but he nevertheless agreed to carry out the experiment. He took a piece of the aorta and of the main leg artery of a dead patient - two locations with characteristically heavy deposits of plaque. I made an incision in the plaques and applied Canesten; the plaques rapidly decomposed. Under the microscope we could see the characteristic threadlike structure of the fungus. The pathologist seemed very surprised, but a few days later he refused to repeat the experiment and was obviously disinclined to associate himself with my radical explanation of the phenomenon.

I then realised that my theory would not easily be accepted. A poorly conducted announcement of my work would probably permanently prevent me from gaining access to medical circles. At that time the Rector of the Medical Academy was Professor Maleev and it was claimed that his position was dependent only on the fact that he was President Zhivkov's brother-in-law. Maleev behaved in the same dictatorial fashion as Zhivkov. The Academy was not in favour of new ideas and my theory was brushed to one side.

Seeking an alternative means of gaining access to the medical establishment I contacted a former classmate who was now a successful heart surgeon. I carefully prepared him and explained the essence of the experiment that I wished him to conduct on my behalf. He advised me to contact a colleague - an assistant lecturer at the department of pathology - and she indeed carried out experiments at my request on atheromatous plaques. She agreed that they confirmed my results but refused to be associated with my theories which she obviously did not take seriously.

As the end of June drew near, Uzunov's daughter suffered a severe attack of asthma and was hospitalized in the Medical Academy. She continued to take 'M' under my direction and I visited her daily in the hospital. A week later her condition improved and she recovered quickly. At the end of the third month of experimenting with 'M' she no longer suffered the attacks that had troubled her previously for several years. I advised her to continue taking 'M' for two further months since when she reported no further attacks.

Uzunov seemed happy but made no comment; not even to express his gratitude. He announced that a biologist working for the Institute of Forensic Medicine would contact me so that we could try to verify my theory. Those were his final words to me; Uzunov never contacted me again about our discussions.

In August I went to the seaside with my son Viktor for a short holiday. The secret service was unable to leave me in peace and agent Protogerov by an extraordinary coincidence occupied the bungalow next to mine in Sozopol from which he greeted me with a friendly smile each day. I was informed that the hospital of the Ministry of the Interior treated diseases not necessarily related to fungoid infections with 'M' just as I had done in my experiments. The drug was now no longer available in the city but Tosho supplied me with a huge quantity. He had no messages for me from his friends and relatives in State Security and claimed that he had not seen them for some time. What was happening to my theory in that great hidden pyramid of power?

At that time I would have given anything to know even a little of what was going on. Uzunov's daughter visited a clairvoyant named Vanga, an old blind woman who had lost her sight in a childhood accident and had subsequently gained a reputation for her extraordinary gift of foretelling the future. She was consulted by thousands and next to her small house in a village near the Greek border was an airfield where her most important visitors, President Zhivkov among them, would regularly arrive for consultation. There was a rumour that even Brezhnev while suffering from cancer of the jaw came from the Kremlin to consult her. Vanga told Uzunov's daughter that she would recover and asked her to tell me that she wanted me to visit her. However I would require a special travel permit to allow me so near to the border and Uzunov refused to issue it. Another five years passed before I eventually visited that remarkable woman. However at the end of the summer of 1980 I could only guess at the events surrounding my work since I was kept completely in the dark.

I assumed that the secret service had thoroughly studied my theory and had sufficient evidence to support it. Quite possibly, experimental work was continuing at the present time but as was normal in such situations all information concerning the outcome of the investigation was considered classified material. I suspect that people at the top of the Ministry of the Interior had decided to support my research and to abandon attempts to force me into joining the secret research institute. I was sure that I was under even closer surveillance than before but at least I was no longer bothered because of my views.

It was possible that the secret service did its best even to convince the dictator Zhivkov that my theory was of importance and that there was a body of evidence to support it; at that time nothing of any import could be made public without his personal approval. It was known that Zhivkov had earlier interfered to support the development of anti-cancer drugs and other new discoveries. In my case however it seemed that his support was going to be difficult to attract. Zhivkov by his very nature was not the man to warm to a radical new theory especially one coming from a known dissident like me. Perhaps Zhivkov's brother-in-law Maleev who himself was a member of the Central Committee of the Communist Party had rejected and ridiculed my theory and its supporters in the secret service. It was only possible for me to guess what went on in a Politburo dominated by family ties and rigid dogma. There was much of which I was inevitably unaware.

In fact I still had no hard evidence that anything to do with my theory was under investigation. The Medical Academy had not replied to my letter and whatever was going on at the lofty summit of communist society would hardly affect my daily life. I still lived in my small attic, Grandmother still supported me and my family constantly worried about the strange effect on me of my medical experimentation.

At the beginning of the year I decided to break up with Tsvete because I expected that I would finally be forced to work for the research institute. She was too young, too reserved and indecisive to cope with my troubles. Beside this she could not understand why I wished to conduct my experiments. I spoke frankly to her telling her of my fears and suggesting that we brought our relationship to an end. She cried and refused to leave me. I felt that I should concentrate more on my scientific work and less on my love affairs. Yet Tsvete stayed with me and began to join me in experimenting with 'M'. Despite her reserve she was eager to help me in any way possible.

Bobby, Shego and I still composed our ridiculous, absurd stories and myths. The hours that I spent with them were the most pleasant of my difficult months of experimentation with 'M'. The three of us would sit on the terrace of a café and obtaining inspiration from the pretty girls passing by, would comment on the power of female beauty and its effect on mere men. Shego continued to be a prolific writer of obscene stories. Sometimes I too would compose a piece with him as the narrator. On one occasion in the café Bobby began to laugh at a story of mine and was unable either to stop or even to get up from his chair while the tears rolled down his cheeks. Shego and I tried to continue reading the story but we laughed too until we collapsed, exhausted. Finally Bobby took the story home with him and told us later that he laughed through the night while trying to read it. Later whenever we remembered that story we continued laughing for hours on end and I remember how much simple laughter helped me at that difficult time.

At the beginning of the autumn a dozen new volunteers agreed with me to start the 'M' therapy. Most were in good health and had little to do beyond hanging around in Shapkite drinking coffee and hoping for something to turn up. It was easy for me to keep a close watch on the progress of the experiments since I spent most of my time there too drinking coffee. One day a new volunteer appeared, a quiet young man with dark hair and pale grey eyes. He said that he was an unemployed graduate in nuclear physics and gave his name as Sergey. I don't think that he even told us his full name or introduced himself properly. I had a very strong feeling that Sergey worked for the secret service but I took him on as a volunteer in the hope that he might be able to tell me what the secret service intended to do with my discoveries.

Soon I was convinced that I was right in my assessment of Sergey. He spent most of his time with me obviously trying to win my confidence. He often carried a briefcase with him and once left it for a short time with me and Tsvete. Thinking that it might be bugged, Tsvete pointed silently to the briefcase and we talked loudly about how much we trusted Sergey. After a time he returned looking extremely pleased and from that moment onward his reactions were an important source of information about what was happening.

A biologist working for the Institute of Forensic Medicine contacted me with an offer to try to find evidence concerning the fungus. After much procrastination we finally made a start on the experiment in one of the laboratories at the University of Sofia. However because the biologist never contacted me again we were unable to conclude the experiment. Sergey once told me that someone, unnamed, had carried out a similar experiment on a tissue culture but I never received official confirmation of it. One day Protogerov announced quietly that I was right to be angry and frustrated because Zhivkov was totally incompetent. This was an extremely dangerous thing for a secret service agent to say. What was he trying to tell me?

Sergey too said that Zhivkov deserved to be shot and hinted that he might know a group of young men who wanted a better future for Bulgaria. He knew that Protogerov was one of them. Sergey told me that he was afraid of the people working for the Department of Safety and Security, the so-called UBO, Zhivkov's personal bodyguards. They had more authority than even the State Security itself and were also empowered to investigate the secret service.

From all these hints and asides I drew the conclusion that the secret service had possibly failed to convince Zhivkov to allow my theory to be made public. Presidential disapproval meant that whatever had begun on 2 April with the treatment of Uzunov's daughter had now come to an end. The secret service considered my discovery to be classified information. There would be no answer from the Medical Academy nor from any other state institute. Nothing would be published about my theory and the experiments surrounding it in Bulgaria or at least, not with my name associated. My future was uncertain, to say the least.

To make sure that I had reached the right conclusion, I telephoned Uzunov and told him of my displeasure because he had broken his word to me. He said nothing. I knew exactly where I stood.

Early one morning at the beginning of December I sat in the deserted *Shapkite* with my traditional cup of nearly-cold coffee, contemplating my future. Here I was, isolated in a small country in the grip of an inflexible communist regime, believing that I had made a fundamental medical discovery which had earned me the personal disfavour of the omnipotent Zhivkov. I faced risks and potential problems in the future which I could not begin to understand. Above all it would be impossible to send information about my discovery to the world outside Bulgaria and the chance of publishing my work abroad now seemed negligible. I felt that the only course available to me - which seemed extremely dangerous - would be to visit foreign embassies in Sofia in the hope of convincing a diplomat to have my theories put to the test in his country.

As I considered this possibility again and again I decided that maybe I should take the risk although it would undoubtedly cause me trouble and might even result in imprisonment or death.

My thirty-seventh birthday was approaching and I had no wish to die. How could I measure the risk? Zhivkov was known to be a dangerous man when his pride was hurt. Having rejected my theory, any visit that I made to a West European embassy could provoke him to order my arrest or even my liquidation. No-one would dare to help me although some people in the secret service obviously supported me. Zhivkov's orders were not to be disobeyed. It was not clear whether I would succeed in persuading a foreign diplomat to forward my article to a research institute abroad. If I failed I might still be arrested simply for visiting an embassy. One thing was certain; I was under surveillance and might be arrested approaching or leaving an embassy if I was so foolish as to make the attempt.

I felt desperately lonely and in my isolation could not rely on anyone to help me. If anything happened to me no-one abroad would ever know anything of my theory and experiments and none of my friends would be able to publish it. I reflected on all those whom I knew. Among them were people working for the secret service who firmly believed my theory but who would do nothing without an order from above. My volunteers conducting the experiment were hardly reliable and most were under surveillance by State Security. Bobby and Shego doubted the validity of my theory and would not join in the experiment. They were my devoted friends but would be powerless if something happened to me. Tsvete would abandon me. My mother believed in me and my grandmother confined to bed by rheumatism, took 'M' and was furious if I overlooked giving her the daily dose. She believed in the treatment, was convinced that it helped her and as usual seemed to be right. Grandmother was well into her eighties but supported me wholeheartedly although she was steadily losing her strength. I wanted to succeed in my work while she was still alive and able to enjoy the fruits of my labours. I desperately hoped that this would happen. Now, more than ten years after his operation for cancer, my father was trying hard to hide the fact that he felt unwell.

I was convinced that because my research could help sick people I should establish contact with some Western embassies at least. This was a hazardous plan but it seemed to be the only one left.

Throughout my life I had taken innumerable risks but nevertheless I felt this time it could be one too many. It was necessary that I should continue my lonely confrontation of a tyrannical system that terrified civilisation as a whole. To improve my chance of success I had only one resource at my disposal and that was courage. I imagined that one day I would succeed, be able to leave Bulgaria, and spend as much time as I liked at the seaside with a beautiful girl in the knowledge that my grandmother was proud of me. For the time being I just had to visit a few Western European embassies.

My first choice was the United States Embassy. The girl receptionist announced my arrival and a fluent Bulgarian-speaking American came to meet me. I immediately felt a chasm opening between us when I asked if the embassy could help me by forwarding my medical research to universities and institutes in the United States. The American official explained courteously that it was forbidden that the embassy should accept any texts, as part of their standing regulations. The embassy's library was at my disposal and if I wished to do so I could look up the addresses of institutes likely to be interested in my work. He informed me however that it was impossible to meet the Cultural Attaché or the Ambassador at this time.

I received the same reception at the British Embassy. Here I was again informed that embassy staff were not allowed to accept material from the local population but the official to whom I spoke offered me a medical magazine in which I could find the addresses of institutes which might be interested to read my paper. I told the official that the Bulgarian postal service was unreliable to say the least and even repeated myself although he seemed to have difficulty in hearing me. Finally I took the magazine and walked away, wondering to myself whether these Western officials realised the risk I took in contacting them.

It was now Christmas and the days passed quietly. I noticed that Sergey had vanished. Perhaps the secret service would now give me the opportunity to incriminate myself by keeping out of range. Then in the first week of January Sergey returned and I told him that my visits to the embassies had been a waste of time. I tried to convince him that I no longer believed that this was the way to publish my research. Soon I returned to my old haunt the Shapkite to drink coffee in the mornings in the company of a few of my volunteers.

On 20 January 1981 Sofia was covered in a thick layer of snow. I packed up my article and made my way to the West German Embassy behind the Borisov Park, near the spot where twenty years ago my jaw had been broken. In my continuing experiments the sores around the old wound looked horrific. Walking in the crunching snow along the quiet narrow streets from the tram stop towards the embassy I had a feeling of euphoria. Something good was about to happen.

At the embassy I asked for the Cultural Attaché. A few moments later a sturdy man in his fifties with grey hair, a beard and spectacles descended the stairs. His name was Rudolf Teske. He spoke English and invited me up to his room on the second floor. I tried to be brief and to the point explaining that I was carrying an important descriptive article on a new therapy to treat a large number of diseases that could not be published in Bulgaria. Teske asked me if I were a medical student. The ice broke as I joked about my age. Teske seemed interested in the drug that I applied in the therapy. I told him that it was well known but he insisted that I should tell him the name.

It seemed that the very word 'M' changed everything immediately.

Teske was silent for a while, fingering his beard. Then he wrote a few notes on a pad and asked me if my article had been offered for publication to any Bulgarian institute. I showed him a copy of the article that I had submitted to the Bulgarian Academy of Science and to the Medical Academy. Teske told me that he knew the chairman of the Academy, Professor Balevski. The article that I gave to him was written in Bulgarian.

Teske asked me if I could provide a translation or summary of the article in German. I said that I would arrange that and suggested that I should return as soon as possible. We decided to meet at the embassy on the following day, 21 January 1981; my thirty-seventh birthday.

Chapter Eleven
Dancing with the Devil

I had very little sleep on the night of my thirty-seventh birthday. At my bedside was a bag containing a German translation of a summary of my theory and copies of the articles that I had sent to the Bulgarian Academy of Science and the Medical Academy and every now and then I looked at them. In the morning on my way to the West German embassy I wondered if I would be able to reach my destination unhindered and every yard ahead of me seemed never-ending. But everything went fine and Teske was awaiting me in his office. After reading the summary and examining the copies of the Bulgarian documents he seemed intrigued and looked up to ask me if I meant all that. Finally he took both the summary and the copies and said that he would do all possible to have the articles examined. I gave him my address and telephone number and left.

Once outside, I felt that a heavy burden had been lifted from my shoulders. I had carefully observed Teske's reactions and had concluded that he could be trusted to hand over my articles to the specialists. I had the distinct impression that Teske knew something about 'M' but how could that be?

The master plan of launching my theory on which the secret service had worked probably included large-scale testing of 'M'. West German pharmaceutical companies had given Bulgaria a licence to produce the drug. Was it now possible that secret service agents were negotiating with those companies to expand production? If so, the question of why Bulgaria was interested in 'M' must have been discreetly asked at the West German embassy and that could explain Teske's reaction. Now West Germany had been provided with the opportunity to examine my research. I could not be absolutely sure but felt that I had found my target.

But it also seemed that I should not push my luck any further. Sergey hinted that I could get into trouble if I continually visited foreign embassies. I felt now that I had made the most of the opportunity and that next time the secret service might draw Zhivkov's attention to me. I therefore pretended that my last visit had been fruitless and said that I could no longer see any point in trying.

After a few months of such contacts, Sergey had become my main source of information. I had no doubt that he worked for the secret service - probably as a member of the special team watching me. That team now seemed to have adopted a strategy differing from the one used in 1976 when Gaydarov and his superiors from State Security had investigated my views.

It seemed obvious to me that the secret service would be displeased with its failure to make my theoretical work public and that it would consider its rejection to be a mistake. However it was impossible to resist the opinion of Zhivkov and the Central Committee of the Communist Party. Nevertheless the secret service quietly tolerated and even supported my experiments with volunteer patients. The team watching included some of the participants in these experiments. Besides Sergey who was probably a trainee in one of the specialised secret service centres, there was a reticent young man - probably his assistant - who hung around carrying a briefcase. He too took 'M'. Special agent Protogerov would logically be part of the team too and Uzunov was undoubtedly among those who were deciding how to deal with me. Possibly there were others and of course the whole operation was closely monitored by high officials in the secret service. There were bugging devices placed all round me and some of the volunteers kicking their heels at the Shapkite were forced to act as informers.

Because of this it was sometimes difficult to bring myself to go to the Shapkite and join in that insane spectacle. But I had no choice; once Teske had taken my articles the only way to maintain touch was by watching those paid to watch me.

My future was uncertain. I suppose that those who dared break the enforced silence by contacting foreign diplomats in Sofia could be counted on the fingers of one hand. Very little was known about them but years later I learned something of the destiny of these people.

At that time Volodya Nakov, a young man of twenty-eight, contacted certain West European embassies to seek their cooperation in his efforts to leave the country. Aided by an Austrian diplomat, he sent letters to the Human Rights conference in Madrid and to Hans-Dietrich Genscher, the West German Foreign Minister, in which he referred to the Helsinki agreement. For that act of defiance Volodya Nakov was sent to prison and was killed in his cell by a psychotic inmate. That is all I know of him; sometimes I think about him and his horrible death appals me.

Then again, Yanko Yankov, a forty year-old scientist working for the Bulgarian Academy of Science, lost his job because of his political views. He made his protest known to certain West European embassies and was then exiled to a small provincial town. He refused however to give up and contacted an American diplomat to ask for his cooperation in leaving the country. For that he received a sentence of twelve years in prison.

The third case of which I know is that of probably the only Bulgarian who actually succeeded in emigrating to the West by making a public protest. After a long prison sentence because of his political views, Dr Nikola Popov published an open letter to Mitterrand in *Le Monde* and went on hunger strike. There was strong public reaction, a committee supporting his case was set up abroad and he was granted freedom in 1982.

However in the winter of 1981 I knew nothing of these men. It was only my intuition that suggested to me I could very well end up like them. I told myself that with a little patience I would be able to learn more about my future. Whatever was in store for me whether good or bad would no longer be hidden from me.

One February morning I met Sergey and his silent assistant in the café. They both sat there with faces frozen as if posing for a picture.

I felt that something had happened.

I engaged Sergey in conversation; studying his reactions. It was not easy to force information from him. I carefully chose my words while provoking him to react. Could it be that Sergey did not realize that he was providing me with the information? Possibly impressed by the situation in which he found himself, he was unable to hide his feelings or was it possible that he did it on purpose? I was unsure, but after a long and devious conversation I could hazard a few guesses.

Probably Teske had inquired at the Ministry of Foreign Affairs about the opinion of the Medical Academy after he had received some positive reactions to my articles. Moreover it seemed that he had tracked my letter to the Medical Academy, but neither the Ministry of Foreign Affairs nor the secret service could come up with a statement; at that time Zhivkov was in Moscow attending a congress of the Soviet Communist Party and everyone had to wait for his reaction.

Once again I decided to visit Teske in an attempt to see whether I had guessed correctly. On my way to the West German embassy I met Tosho. On the spur of the moment I decided to invite him to come with me. It would be a daring move demonstrating to the secret service that I could rely on support from abroad. Besides, Teske would see for himself that I was under surveillance and in desperate need of help. Tosho would suit both purposes well; he did not understand a word of English and looked exactly like a KGB agent from a James Bond movie.

Teske looked very pleased with himself and enthusiastic but did not believe me when I introduced Tosho as my associate. Teske explained that he had sent my documents to the Max Planck Institute to be further examined. He assured me that he would do everything necessary to let me know the result. This was all I needed to hear and I shook Teske's hand and left accompanied by Tosho who continued to stare blankly at the wall. It was now obvious to me that something had happened.

Above all it seemed that I had finally succeeded in breaking out of the isolation of my existence. Now my research was being examined by specialists in West Germany and what was more, Teske's attitude showed that the first reactions were positive.

Although Teske mentioned nothing, he had most probably contacted the Bulgarian authorities about me. That would mean that my case was on the agenda of diplomatic relations between West Germany and Bulgaria. At the time West Germany was Bulgaria's principal trading partner in the West and had developed a relaxed and pragmatic foreign policy (the *Ostpolitik*) towards communist countries. West German diplomacy had acquired much experience from its relations with the East German regime and had discreetly arranged for many thousands of political prisoners to cross the border to the West. Since great tact was an important feature of West German policy, my case would be treated discreetly and Teske's reluctance to provide me with the information was not surprising. What would his intervention mean for me?

I now seemed to have a unique opportunity to radically change my life. I believed that the results of my research would be confirmed in West Germany and despite the revolutionary nature of its implications, would be published abroad. Not for one second did I imagine that my theories would fail to be recognized in the West. In my mind whatever the Bulgarian authorities intended to do in the near future, matters would soon change and one day the world would take notice of me and my theories.

These conclusions gave me much satisfaction but they also implied that I would have no influence on what was going to happen and moreover I would be constantly kept in the dark. The single source of information available to me was Sergey. In those days he always took that little briefcase with him wherever he went. He was very curious about everything and our conversations while drinking coffee in the morning resembled passages from a spy novel. Sergey's interest in my recent visit to the West German embassy was as great as my eagerness to know what the Bulgarian authorities intended to do. I was impatient to learn their reaction to the West German interference.

A few weeks later I had the impression that Sergey brought news for me. From our cryptic conversation I managed to get a hint of what the Ministry of Foreign Affairs had said about me to Teske: I was declared mentally ill and my theories were born of insanity. From long conversations with Sergey in the following days I managed to learn what the West Germans in turn thought of me. It appeared that they did not consider me insane. Beside my research on the fungus they had referred to my engine patent as proof of sanity.

In my thoughts I thanked Teske, wondering how he had come to know about the engine. Then I thought of the other holder of a private patent, my investor Stoyan Cholakov, who had also visited foreign embassies although which I knew not. I visited him immediately. He told me that he had visited Teske in the previous year and had told him of his patent and mine, mentioning BMW's interest in my invention. His visit had little effect except to generate trouble with the secret service. Finally I had a reaction. I had given up with the idea that one day my engine would see daylight but now it seemed that there was still a possibility of arousing interest.

I based my speculation about the possible discussions between Teske and the Bulgarian authorities concerning my case only on what I had learned from Sergey. I had no idea whether I could rely on his patchy information and until the end of March I heard nothing new. However Sergey persuaded me to visit Teske again from which I concluded that the secret service was eager to learn about the next step that West German diplomacy might take to press my case.

I was equally eager. In April I once more visited the West German embassy and Teske told me there was no news for me. He said that he was very busy as he had much to do in preparing for the Bulgarian cultural week in West Germany. I pointed out that I had problems in Bulgaria and wished to leave for West Germany. His reaction to my expressed wish was rather subdued.

At the beginning of May, forming part of the festivities for the thirteenth centenary of the founding of the Bulgarian State, a cultural week was organised in Hamburg. Teske had done much indeed. In the newspapers I read about a whole week of symposia, exhibitions, concerts, movies, radio and TV programmes on Bulgaria. The opening was attended by the Chancellor's wife and other prominent functionaries. Among Bulgarian representatives I noted the names of Angel Balevski, Chairman of the Bulgarian Academy of Science and Milcho Germanov, Deputy Chairman of the Committee for Culture.

Milcho Germanov was Shego's uncle.

I asked Shego whether he could arrange for me to meet him. A few days later I was invited to Milcho Germanov's office. He was a wary *apparatchik,* but still provided me with some information. It was not necessary for me to ask because Milcho Germanov demonstrated a spontaneous interest in my research. I had no doubt that his West German hosts had brought up the subject of my work in Hamburg. I had the feeling that something seemed to have been published on the subject but he would not tell me what. Although the West Germans had put in a good word for me the chairmen and deputies of the Bulgarian academies and committees were not impressed. They reported to their party bosses and obediently carried out orders. Despite his personal interest in my case Milcho Germanov refrained from making any commitment.

At last I felt that I had proof that West Germany had made discreet but nevertheless serious efforts to promote my case with the Bulgarian authorities. Clearly that could have only been done because the Max Planck Institute had reacted positively to my research. It was also obvious to me that West Germany had supported my case from desire for cooperation and in order to maintain good relations despite the hostility of the Bulgarian authorities towards me.

I decided to speak to Teske again. Now he seemed more mysterious than ever before. I told him that I had heard that something about my research had appeared in West Germany. Teske asked how I knew that and I told him about my meeting with Milcho Germanov. At this Teske looked inquisitively at me and after hesitating confirmed the news.

It seemed that there was nothing else that he could tell me and in fact he expected to hear more from me. I explained that I was in a difficult situation and insisted on being permitted to leave for West Germany. Teske said nothing beyond confirming that he would try to let me know what had been published. He promised to contact me when there was more news but now clearly wished to avoid further face to face contact; preferring to be left alone to see what he could do to help me.

I naturally concluded that Teske had good reasons for acting in that way and that it was probably necessary for me to accept the situation if the West Germans were to help me. It seemed that the West German foreign office had taken my case seriously and there was nothing more that I could do to influence the situation.

Outside in the street Sergey and the entire invisible army of the secret service awaited me. Sergey had offered me the chance of earning a lot of money by agreeing to carry a miniature tape-recorder during my visits to the West German embassy. However I had refused to listen to him - there may have been no bugging devices in the embassy but there were certainly enough of them around me.

After all the fuss about the festivities in Hamburg and the rumours of the publication of my research there followed a period of total silence. I was able to learn nothing about the reaction to events of the Bulgarian authorities. On the contrary, it seemed that I was expected to provide Sergey with information.

Then on a July morning I read in the newspaper that the West German Foreign Minister Hans-Dietrich Genscher was soon to visit Bulgaria. The news of this visit was astonishing.

In the summer of 1981 Western civilization was faced by overwhelmingly powerful Soviet military supremacy. Soviet missiles could destroy Europe in a matter of minutes and the communist land armies clearly outmatched Western defence forces. The ideological paranoia and the economic impotence of the communist system led by the demented Soviet party chiefs could bring the world to nuclear war. Faced with such potential blackmail, West European countries accepted the need to deploy American mid-range missiles on their territory. This action provoked a volte-face in communist policy; relations with the West were frozen and the hysterical campaign of propaganda was launched. As always, Bulgaria was the most zealous participant in this campaign which no longer welcomed Western European foreign ministers. How was it that the Sofia regime, notorious for its Soviet-dominated foreign policy, now attracted the attention of the West German Foreign Minister?

I wondered whether my case was part of Genscher's agenda. After a few months of attempted intervention, the West German diplomats had probably reached the conclusion that it would not be easy to negotiate my case with the Bulgarian authorities. I was known to be an outcast. In such cases however it was West German policy never to seek confrontation but discreetly to seek a solution by maintaining good relations through offers of cooperation and economic help. My clearly stated intention to Teske to leave Bulgaria probably gave Genscher the opportunity to reach an agreement.

In the days leading up to the visit I heard Sergey say amazing things. He asked me earnestly whether I would be willing to accept West German citizenship. At that I laughed - could anyone honestly imagine that I would not? But the question itself suggested that my case was possibly on the visit agenda and after my conversation with Sergey I reached the conclusion that the authorities were considering whether to allow me to leave for West Germany. What were the other possibilities? Hardly any of the people with whom Genscher would be obliged to negotiate on my behalf would be willing to wave goodbye to me at the airport.

On 8th August Genscher arrived in Sofia for a two-day visit. On the following day he departed for the governmental residence in Varna where it was intended that he would negotiate with his Bulgarian counterpart, Mladenov.

Sergey and I took a long walk through the streets of Sofia in the pleasantly warm evening air of the day before Genscher left. Sergey had left his briefcase behind and as we stood alone on the pavement of the Vitoshka Boulevard he suddenly said very quietly that the Bulgarian authorities had signed an agreement with West Germany to cooperate on the development of my engine. That night I lay awake, wondering what might happen next.

On the following morning I was picked up by two heavies outside my door and pushed into a plain Lada without explanation. Their silence was absolute but the mystery was soon explained; I was taken to the interrogation department of State Security where Inspector Lyubomir Kotsev awaited me. He was the same inspector who had been in charge of the investigation of Lyubo Kanov three years before.

Assisted by a lady officer, Kotsev began to cross-examine me about my experiments with 'M' on volunteers. Finally he took out the criminal code and read to me an article forbidding all illegal practice of medicine. He said that it provided him with grounds to begin an investigation and I assumed that he was using this as an argument to subject me to pressure. His intentions then became clear when he announced that I could choose between either being arrested for preliminary investigation or signing a statement that I would cease my visits to the West German embassy. I signed the statement. Then Kotsev insisted that I should see a psychiatrist and rambled on to admit that he personally approved my medical theories which he found intriguing.

I walked home reflecting on what had happened. My initial conclusion was that my case had been discussed during Genscher's meetings with his Bulgarian counterpart Mladenov. Wasn't it the case that the authorities intended to keep me in the dark about these talks by forcing me to sign an undertaking not to visit the embassy? Regardless of this, the manner in which Inspector Kotsev had insisted that I should see a psychiatrist told me that I was in for trouble.

I was not mistaken. On the same day Sergey insisted that I should begin working on the engine and told me that my fungus research in West Germany had not been published. He also informed me that one of the regular Shapkite customers, a strange-looking bearded man, was known to be seeking revenge for some personal reason and might possibly beat me up. Indeed this man began to telephone me to make threats. Sergey seemed to be unaffected by his change in attitude to me. In past months I had attempted to discover what his views were and he told me once that the most important objective was to eliminate man's exploitation of man. With such views he would undoubtedly carry out any order from his superiors without a moment's hesitation. Therefore it was not difficult to conclude that Genscher's visit had radically changed things for me.

Above all the secret service was now working on me in a new and more aggressive way. Their obvious intention was as two years ago, to force me into working for a major secret institute by blackmail and manipulation. My engine had become the means of increasing pressure on me and my research on the fungus was now under attack. What was the reason for this?

At the time it was very difficult for me to obtain any reliable information; even Sergey would say nothing and behaved like an automaton. I based my speculation on the last piece of information given to me by Sergey - that an agreement to develop my engine had been signed during Genscher's visit.

I tried to consider what were the motives of the West Germans in attempting to seek an agreement affecting me. Most possibly the West German diplomats had decided that they were not in a position to judge my provocative theory in the medicinal field especially after the reluctance of the Bulgarian authorities to do so and their conviction that I needed the attention of a psychiatrist.

Perhaps medical specialists had reacted positively to my research and that is why the diplomats were now willing to find a solution for my difficult situation. However the acceptance of a revolutionary medical theory was something for medical experts rather than for diplomats. In the impasse created by the rigid position of the Bulgarian authorities, I assumed that the West German diplomats preferred to use my engine invention rather than the fungus theory as their argument in the negotiations. I could not believe that the engine alone was sufficiently interesting to attract the attention of the diplomatic service. However it might seem a way for West Germany to come to an agreement about me although their main interest lay in my research on the fungus.

It was much more difficult to surmise what might be the intention of the Bulgarian authorities. Those people who had kept me in isolation and under surveillance day and night by secret agents and bugging devices had now begun a new campaign of repression and manipulation in order to force me into accepting whatever it was they had decided to do with me. Their motivation and manner of thinking were the result of ideological paranoia and I could see no logic in their behaviour. To them West Germany and Western civilization in general were mortal enemies and any influence from abroad was treated with total hostility. By seeking an agreement to cooperate in my case aroused suspicion of hostility on the part of West Germany and interest shown in my engine aroused speculation that the West was interested to acquire my intellect for the war of advance technologies on their side. This manner of thinking was typical of the secret service and was how the ideological struggle experts and the Quiet Front worked to isolate Bulgaria from the rest of Europe while supporting terrorists and their activities.

Perhaps at the time the senior Party hierarchy was prepared to let me leave for West Germany if only to wash their hands of the whole affair; this could have been the reason why foreign minister Mladenov had signed the agreement. I suspected the hand of the secret service in all of this with its desire to maintain the situation under its direct control. At that time the secret service was more influential than any other element of the administrative structure of the country. Mladenov would hardly bother to maintain his side of the agreement. Years later for example, after the fall of Zhivkov and in the face of the first spontaneous demonstration in Sofia, the same Mladenov this time as President of Bulgaria, yelled `send for the tanks'!

It seemed clear that the secret service had decided to keep me in the dark about the agreement and to consequently block it or even sink it. Most probably the service thought that the West Germans were motivated by their interest in my engine and not by my research on the fungus. Could it be that obsessed by my engine, the secret service were scheming on how they could profit from my rights to the patent? In one way or the other it was obvious to me that on this occasion I would be forced by all possible means into agreeing to work on the engine at the secret state institute.

As I considered all that I realised that those plotting under the cover of secrecy to harass me were anything but altruistic; on the other hand they were excessively paranoid and perhaps even stupid. Would I be able to resist the treatment they were preparing for me?

Soon I became convinced that my conclusions were correct. In the weeks ahead Sergey acted clearly in a manner suggesting that he was following new instructions to press me into agreeing to work on the engine at the secret institute. Under the same instructions, agent Protogerov pretended to bump into me in the street and reminded me that I should see a psychiatrist while the bearded customer of the Shapkite whom I had insulted in some mysterious way of which I was unaware resumed calling me regularly to threaten me in a melodramatic manner.

Besides Sergey and the secret service agents, there were others engaged to blackmail and manipulate me. Some of my volunteers confessed that they had been forced by the secret service to ask me about certain things and to then report on my response. A friend of mine whose father worked for State Security said that she was sent to see me and was later interrogated by secret service agents. Stoyan Cholakov had withdrawn part of his investment in my patent, leaving me a loan that I had to pay back to a man from Plovdiv. That man and his loan soon turned out to be instruments for applying further pressure on me. At the same time attempts were made to turn Tsvete and Bobby into informers on behalf of the secret service. By the end of August more than ten people in my circle were actually engaged in manipulating me into working for the secret institute.

I then decided to approach Milcho Germanov. Once again he received me and expressed interest in my research about which I had prepared a summary for him. The Committee for Culture of which he was deputy chairman was headed by Zhivkov's daughter Lyudmila Zhivkova. She was known to be a neurotic woman strongly attracted to Buddhism and mystic cults. Zhivkov, whose son had become an alcoholic, determined to appoint his daughter as his successor and openly promoted her career in the Party ranks with limitless powers. Thus I felt that there was nothing I could lose by seeking the support of the Committee for Culture. Could this be a way to avoid the blackmail of the Secret Service?

However it was not Lyudmila Zhivkova but Colonel Christozko Uzunov who instructed me to report to the Lenin Police Department. As I entered Uzunov's room I knew by the evil look on his face that he was not going to thank me for helping his daughter. It was obvious to me that Uzunov had finally lost patience. His efforts to force me into working for the secret institute had had no result so far. Possibly he was infuriated by the synopsis I had given to Milcho Germanov and had decided to personally set things straight with me. He began to yell at me, saying that I was insane. He branded my research on the fungus as the work of a madman and even declared that the West German embassy had lodged a complaint against me. I had not yet seen a psychiatrist as had been ordered and he now gave me a three-day ultimatum to do so. Finally Uzunov revealed his hand by stating that all my troubles were the result of my refusal to work for the secret institute. It seemed that he was the originator of the pressure on me and was anxious to see results. Uzunov insisted that I should immediately withdraw my synopsis from Milcho Germanov and in the end he warned me that if I ever intended to write a book about my experiences I must not claim that I had been persecuted, as that was untrue.

It was obvious that there was only one matter on which Uzunov and I agreed and that was the book that I should write one day. I ignored his threats and left his office asking myself whether he had ever been personally embarrassed by his insolence. It was obvious that the power he held and his ambition to break my resistance by blackmail put me into a difficult situation. Uzunov seemed obsessed and he was in a position to easily order my submission after the three-day ultimatum; most possibly by not declaring my arrest publicly.

I found myself at an impasse. The secret service would prevent me from making any further visits to the West German embassy but in any case there was very little the Germans could do to help me. Neither Milcho Germanov nor any other person in Bulgaria could interfere with the secret service. At that time no-one even dared to protest about its heavy-handedness. I once saw an agent in plain clothes strike a young man on the head with his pistol butt while stunned spectators silently stood around. On the following day at about five o'clock in the afternoon Tsvete, Bobby and I went to the Havana café. I told them how desperate I was and Bobby agreed that very little could be done and that only God could help me now. At that very moment I saw Teske enter the Havana in the company of a lady, probably his wife. They came towards us looking for a free table. Teske noticed me and approached to introduce me to his wife and to ask how I was. Then they sat at a table next to ours while I noticed a secret service agent in plain clothes and sandals approach in order to listen to the conversation. There was a look of plain bewilderment on his face as he stood near our table for a while.

That chance meeting had certainly changed things for me.

I had received a few strokes of good luck in my life. In 1961 there was a power cut at the very moment that my interrogators prepared to beat me up in my prison cell. My chance meeting with Teske was pure luck but no-one in the secret service would believe that. In their paranoid minds nothing happened by chance and they always suspected some larger motive behind everything.

Indeed during that same evening I noticed that the secret service was in a state of high alarm. Sergey appeared immediately and was restless, stirring in his seat and muttering that something very strange had happened. In the end he announced that he was impressed by the West German intelligence service and thought that someone high up in the Bulgarian hierarchy had given them information. It was not only Sergey who behaved like a madman.

The heroes of the Quiet Front were obviously closing in on me and were escorting me as I walked through the streets as though I were an Oriental potentate. In the evening a couple of heavies stood at the entrance to my flat. On the following morning they were there, freshly shaven, patient and determined as ever. I took a ride in Shego's car and noticed that a black Volga followed us closely all the time.

Undoubtedly I had been under twenty-four hour surveillance before but now the situation assumed unrealistic proportions. It was clear that the secret service would do anything to prevent me from making public statements and they must have suspected me of being secretly in touch with Teske. I therefore decided to take advantage of their baseless fears and told Sergey that Teske would be informed if I were subjected to further harassment. This was a blatant lie and two days later when I chanced to see Teske in the City Garden he did not even notice me. Nevertheless, Uzunov did not call again.

In those days I would often sit alone in the city garden on the terrace of a small café near the Congo corner where we used to play as children. There I could peacefully reflect on life. The end of summer was drawing near and I realised that my life had become dangerous in recent months. The events in which I was caught up seemed to restrict my small chances of ever receiving a permit to travel abroad and I felt that I could easily be arrested. So far the communist regime had prevented any of my activities from becoming public. Because of the confidential character of the diplomatic interference my name was suppressed. Possibly contingency plans had been prepared for use if my case became public. Could these include an attempt on my life?

During the year and a half that I had experimented with 'M' I had progressively lost hope of receiving any support for my research in Bulgaria. After recent events I warned my volunteers that in the future I would be unable to monitor experiments with others and was no longer able to advise on the correct daily dose of 'M'. Still I had compiled sufficient evidence from my observations and was able to elaborate my theory.

The evidence obtained confirmed the ideas that I had formed during the first months of experimentation. Several cycles could be observed in my own curative crises as well as in those of the volunteers. One of them took twenty-four hours with a deterioration peak at the same hour, after which dead cells peeled off. Another cycle continued for a period of several months, gradually peaking and then subsiding. The effect could easily be observed on the skin and I concluded that the fungi located at different places in the body were connected by a single organism known in biology as a heterokaryon. In a heterokaryon a number of fungi are connected by a common network and individual cell walls are open allowing the protoplasm to form a common liquid environment in which cell nuclei move around freely. In the heterokaryon many cells form hollow fibres with thick walls. In decaying dead tissue I found fibres ten inches long with the diameter of a thin hair. Peeling off a piece of tissue from the skin would sometimes cause a detachment of tissue elsewhere in the body, probably because a common heterokaryon was being torn apart. At that point I asked myself a couple of questions: it was known that the protoplasm of some fungi contained viruses which influenced their mutation and made them more viable. Could it be that viruses moved without obstruction in the protoplasm of heterokaryons developing in the human body? Could it be that the viruses themselves were the instrument by which fungus attacked human tissue? Could it be that viruses were part of the fungi and their strange way of life?

I was unable to provide an answer to these questions at this time but I continued to analyse what I felt during the curative crises. Most of them reminded me of old illnesses, mainly connected with my sinusitis and my stomach. I also felt sensations that did not resemble anything so far experienced; sometimes the effects were frightening and overwhelming. At times my blood pressure would rise to 220/110 and I would feel faint, possibly because huge quantities of dead tissue were being discarded in my blood vessels. In general the effects of the experiment were unpleasant but I felt that they led to a gentle improvement in my health. Others among the forty people of all ages taking part in my experiment had similar experiences. During the several months when I observed them, most did not experience a heavy curative crisis. Only one of them ended up with fluid in his lungs requiring hospitalization to have them drained. Previously he had suffered from an extended lung infection and therefore withdrew from the experimental process. From observation of my younger volunteers I concluded that after a period of a year or so the process of rejecting dead tissue continued automatically without the need to take 'M'. That meant that the immune system had taken over the process.

More recently my ideas on human biology progressively diverged from mainstream thought. I imagined that the heterokaryon, that monstrous fungoid web buried in dead tissue, was an enormous invisible being living within the human organism. By taking over more and more tissue with the onset of old age, the heterokaryon probably caused many changes in the body. Was not ageing skin a manifestation of that process and perhaps similar changes took place in other tissues too, mainly in the blood vessels? The deposition of dead tissue could easily be seen in any part of the human body; for example the female hand mercilessly betrays its age.

Approaching these ideas made me appreciate the huge chasm between my beliefs and current medical thought. Although the fungus had a simple structure, no-one, not even science fiction writers, had so far suspected its existence. I contemplated the belief of God and the devil inhabiting the human universe, engaged in an eternal struggle. Doesn't the fungus remind us of the Devil with his drooping old man's nose?

Although I was pleased to be able to elaborate my theory, I felt disappointed that I was unable to use modern technology in my continuing research into the facts that I had discovered. I believed that I had succeeded in drawing others into examining my discovery yet there was still one problem; the experiment that I had carried out made it impossible to seek the help of medical experts. What had taken place in my body contradicted modern medicinal methods. For example I expected that if I were to lose consciousness because of a sudden rise of blood pressure I would be treated with a drug that would lead to the formation of clots in my blood vessels.

The only thing I could do was to use 'M' and my courage to fight the Devil if the fungus really symbolized him. That did not seem easy in my situation but once I had begun there was no reason why I should stop before reaching a conclusion. I said to myself that from now on the risk would not disappear but nor would it change very much either.

It was difficult to believe that I took such a huge risk. In September I found a job as an artist painting restaurant signs for a tiny salary. Only Tsvete, Bobby and Shego remained with me.

There was Sergey of course from whom I attempted to draw hints of what the future held for me. I had already made it clear that I understood his part in my harassment but that did not seem to bother him. The last piece of information I squeezed out of him was about a possible agreement with West Germany of which I awaited the results. The conclusion was now obvious; the Bulgarian authorities had no intention of keeping their part of it.

It seemed that the secret service had accepted that I preferred to paint sign boards rather than work for the secret institute. This was a kind of trench warfare with the authorities waiting to see how the West German diplomats would react to the Bulgarian refusal to implement my engine agreement. In fact if the Bulgarians refused to capitulate and prevented me from leaving the country the only possibility left for me was to wait until the publication of my fungus research and reactions to it. That is of course unless I decided to do something about the situation.

Although I was still kept under tight surveillance I continued to believe that the involvement of the diplomatic services granted me some kind of immunity. The hysterical reaction of the secret service to my chance meeting with Teske proved this to me. Now I could not gain anything by contacting the embassy but I anticipated that by the end of the year West Germany would raise the matter of the failure by Bulgaria to implement the agreement. There was much uncertainty in my speculation which meant that I could not fully appreciate the risk I was taking. But risk had become part of my daily life and to continue taking risks was the only way in which I could change my situation.

Just before Christmas I lost my job as a sign printer. Tsvete came to see me in my attic in the evening and I told her that I would go on hunger strike unless I was allowed to leave the country. The bugging devices installed in my tiny room conveyed the message to the authorities.

This was the beginning of my thirteenth attempt to leave the country.

Chapter Twelve
Wiesbaden

I ushered in 1982 by lying on the hard bed of my cold attic on hunger strike. I wished to express my resistance to the suffocating grip of State Security around me, since I could no longer tolerate the row of puppets lined up outside the house headed by Sergey each time that I walked out. It was time to demonstrate to the manipulators that I was not prepared to accept their interference in my life.

However, what was happening remained completely invisible to the outside world. No one knew that Western diplomats had interfered in my situation or that I had gone on hunger strike with the risk of further serious repression. Only Tsvete came to see me each day to share my problems. I had told Bobby and Shego too, but only saw them occasionally.

The hunger strike was not a pleasant experience. Starvation is sometimes applied as a therapy and its effects are similar to the curative crises resulting from a course of 'M'. My hunger strike intensified the working of the drug on my body and by the end of the second week I felt thoroughly exhausted.

Shortly before 20th January the press announced that on that day the Bulgarian Foreign Minister Mladenov would again meet his West German counterpart, Genscher. It was now exactly a year since I had visited the West German embassy. Could this be the long- anticipated response by West Germany to Bulgaria's failure to perform their agreement about my fate? When the news reached me I was well into the fourth week of starvation. On that very same day the telephone threats resumed to inform me that I would be beaten up if I dared to leave my room. This was the Bulgarian authorities' and the secret service's reaction to my situation which now seemed highly unpleasant.

It was naive of me to imagine that my work on fundamental medical research could secure the respect of the authorities. The communist regime was not known for its good manners but as a propaganda machine worked assiduously to present a refined and cultured veneer to the outside world. The threats against me that had been issued because of my reluctance to cooperate with the secret service demonstrated clearly that I was at the mercy of desperate villains with unbounded cynicism and cruelty. I was convinced that these people were quite prepared to carry out their threats to beat me up.

All in all, I seemed to be in a nasty situation.

Physical violence was the favourite method of the Bulgarian communist regime when dealing with opponents. The police systematically physically abused arrested suspects and it was common practice to assault anyone who deviated from communist standards of behaviour. State Security agents were trained and instructed to use physical force; many of them obviously enjoyed their work. It was unwise to attempt to lodge a complaint after maltreatment and from its very beginning until well into 1989 the regime held the population in a tight physical grip. After the collapse of the system the State Security professional thugs organised into mafia-like groups that continued to terrorise their fellow

Bulgarians with even greater brutality. Associating with the hardliners, they maintained their power, influence and organisation and forced the country into ever-worsening crisis during the following seven years. It was not before the spring of 1997 that the communists finally relinquished the power that they could no longer maintain by the use of violence even against members of the public; even those on a hunger strike.

My jaw, fractured in 1961, was very helpful to me in my experiment with 'M' while providing much evidence. Nevertheless I was not eager to be beaten up again and such an experience would solve none of my problems. The secret service could easily arrange for me to be attacked without me being able to prove anything. In the previous year I had gone to the local policeman to complain about the telephone threats. He had ignored my complaint and cynically suggested that I should contact Colonel Uzunov, the very man who had threatened to arrest me if I did not consult a psychiatrist.

It seemed to me that I had reached a dangerous point in my protest against State Security manipulation. Anything that I might do, even discontinuing my futile hunger strike, could bring on further repression intended to force me into the role planned for me by the secret service. Having taken all that into consideration I decided that the only chance to gain my freedom would be to give in to the threats. If anything could help me it would be fear on the part of the regime that it could be discredited if my case became public knowledge. Its hysterical reaction to my chance meeting with Teske supported me in this belief.

I analysed the intimidation applied to me. Beyond physical violence I had been threatened with committal to a psychiatric clinic. This was not the idea of anonymous callers but of state officials; investigator Lyubomir Kotsev, the state security head of the Lenin department Colonel Christozko Uzunov and his subordinate agent Slavcho Protogerov. All three had demanded in their official capacity that I should see a psychiatrist. If they could arrange for me to be committed to a psychiatric hospital as was regularly done with dissidents in the Soviet Union they would surely do it without a moment's hesitation. Was it perhaps not time for me to comply with their demands? At this time my hospitalization in a psychiatric clinic would create more problems for those willing to manipulate me while complaints as a result of being beaten would hardly concern them. Anyway these people would not give up until they were convinced that I was ready to pay any price for my freedom.

Following this line of thought I realised that I could escape from the present nightmare either by entering a psychiatric clinic or by accepting a position at the secret research institute. The latter would entail becoming a servant of the criminals who terrorised me.

It was now two days before my thirty-eighth birthday and I wished that I had a third option. At the present time it seemed that the psychiatric clinic was my best choice. If my speculation was right my blackmailers would be thwarted in their plans by my admission to hospital. I was not the only one who believed that my work might become publicly known in the West. The secret service shared this conviction, too. It probably did not think that I happened to go on a hunger strike on the very day that West German diplomats reacted to the situation. It was essential to sustain the authorities' fear that my case could become public, or else I knew that I was lost. At the moment my only trump card was the potential embarrassment of the Bulgarian

At work in my attic

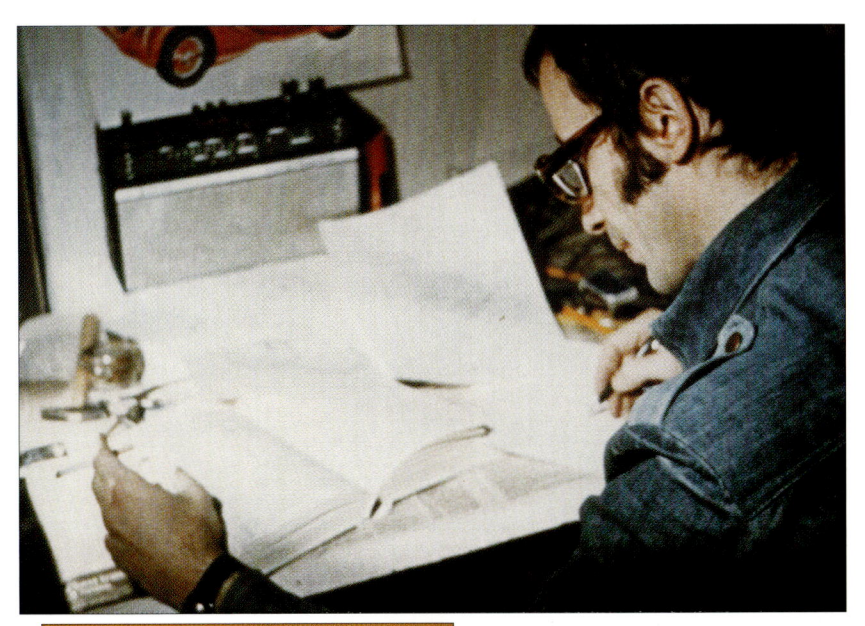

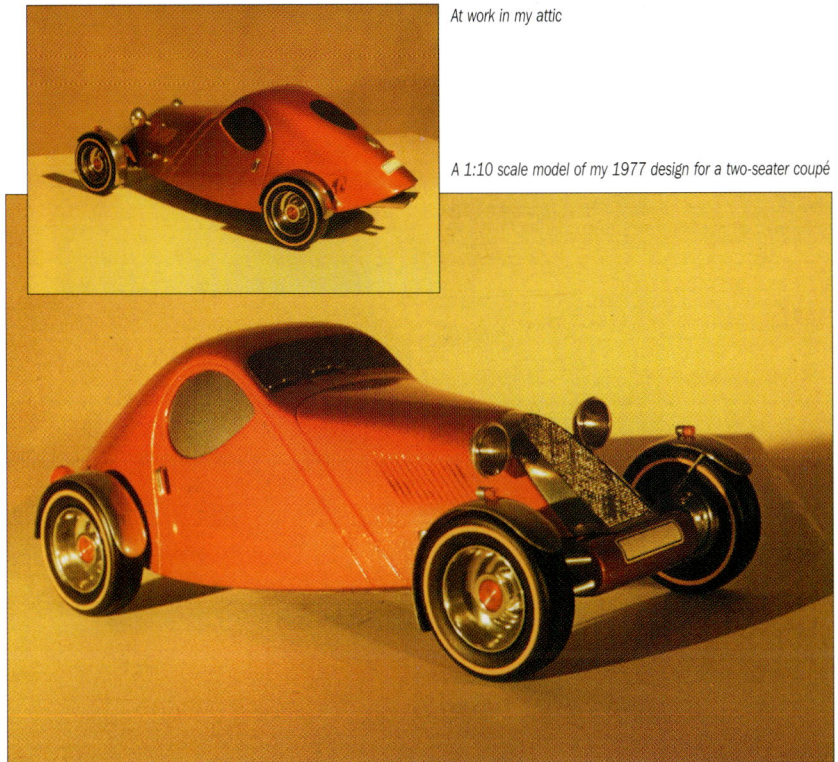

A 1:10 scale model of my 1977 design for a two-seater coupé

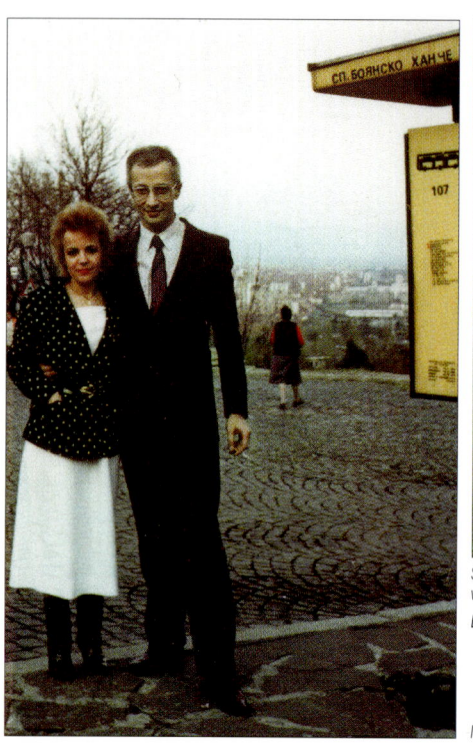

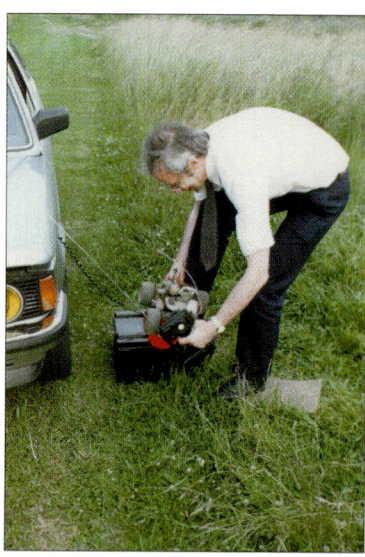

Starting the motor of the radio-controlled model car fitted with my gearbox

Edith and I at the bus stop in Boyana (left)

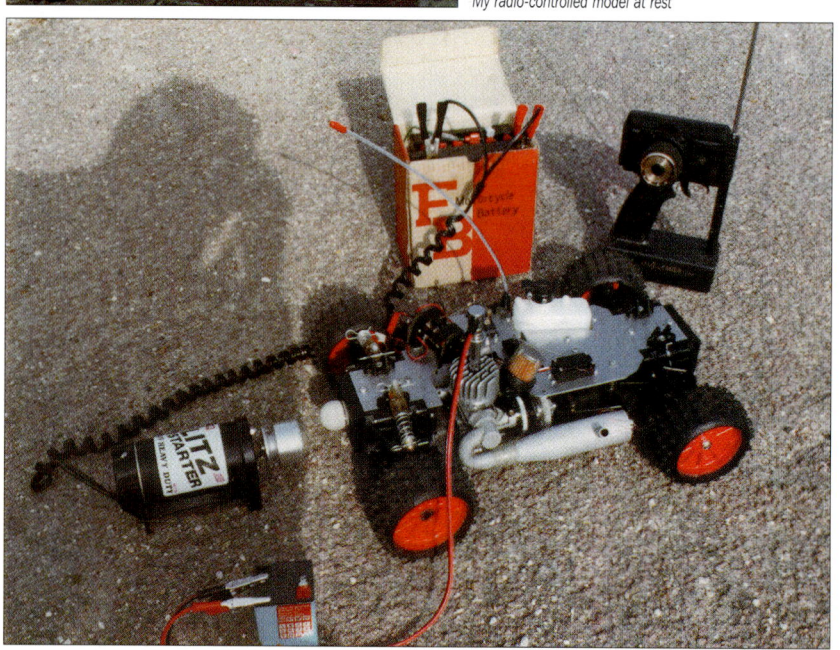

My radio-controlled model at rest

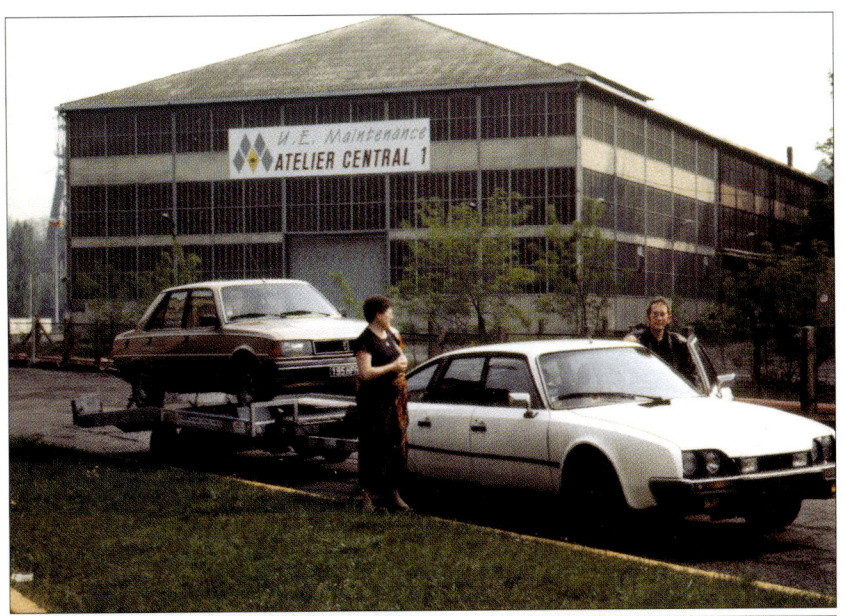

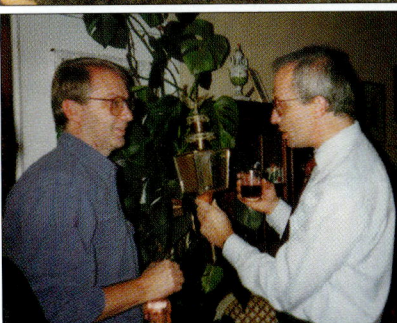

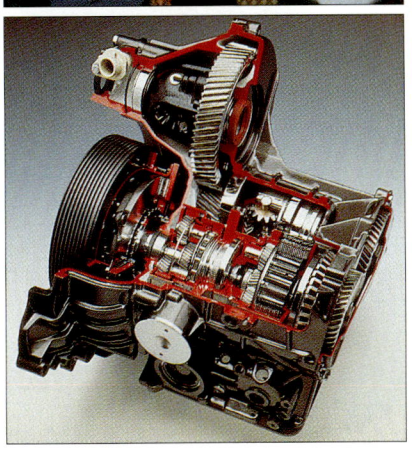

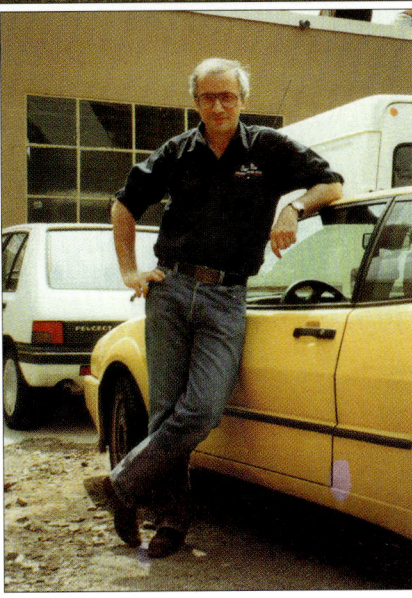

Pierrot and his wife ready to trail away from the mines' mechanical workshop in Petite-Rosselle the Peugeot 305 fitted with my transmission

The Antonov automatic transmission

With Dan Wysenbeek, the Dutchman who suggested we found a company in Rotterdam

In front of the workshop at Petite-Rosselle

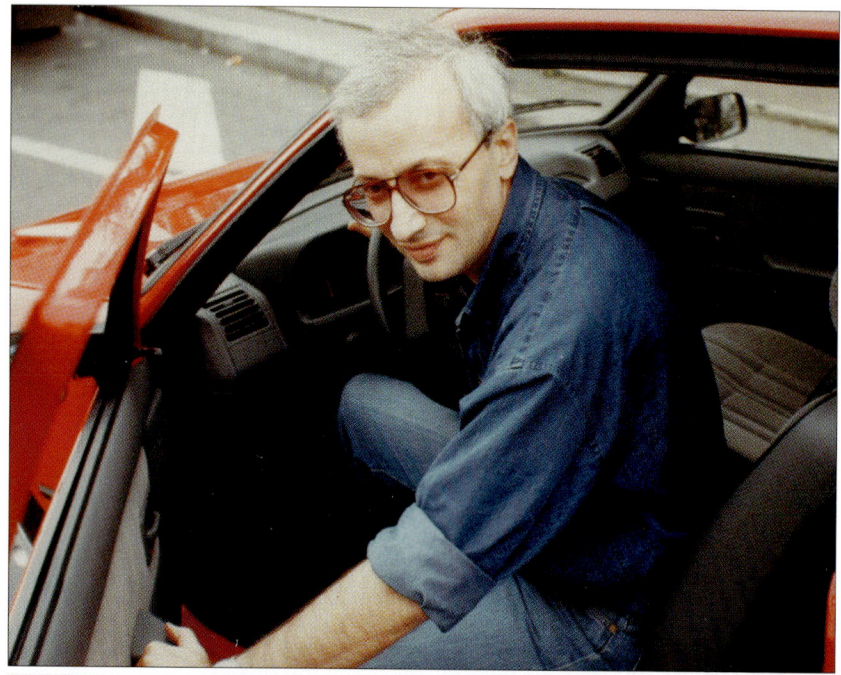

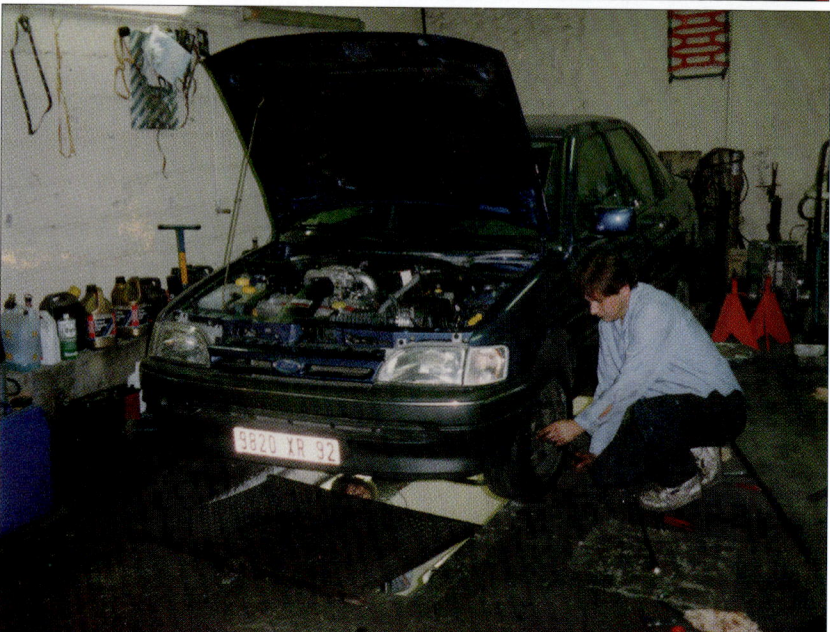

In a Peugeot 205 fitted with one of the new prototype Antonov automatic transmissions

Jean-Claude completing assembly of a prototype transmission

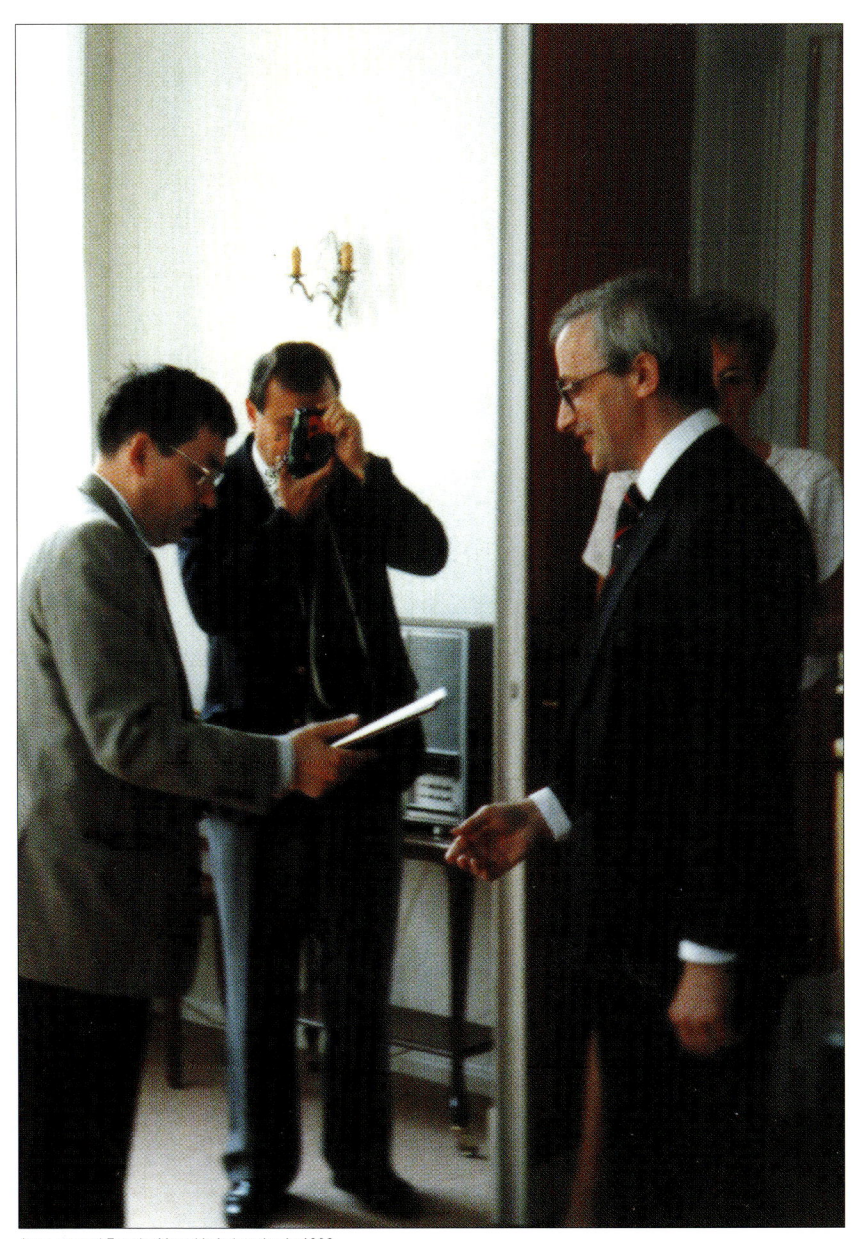

I was granted French citizenship in Lorraine in 1993

In Tokyo, 1993

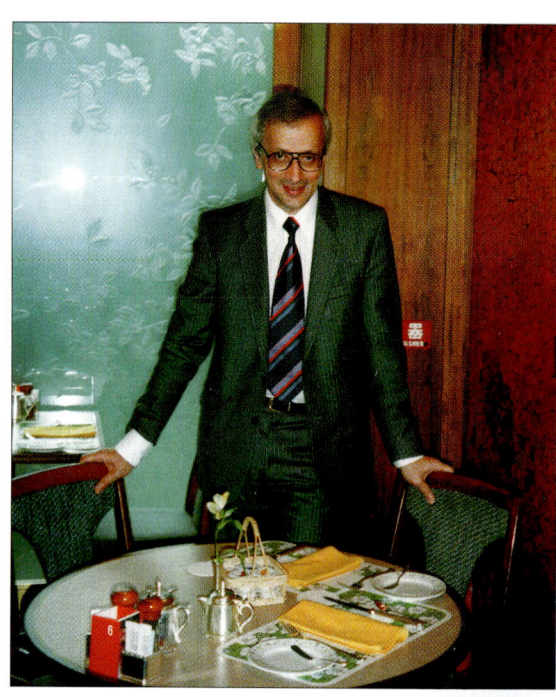

Testing the prototype of my engine in 1996

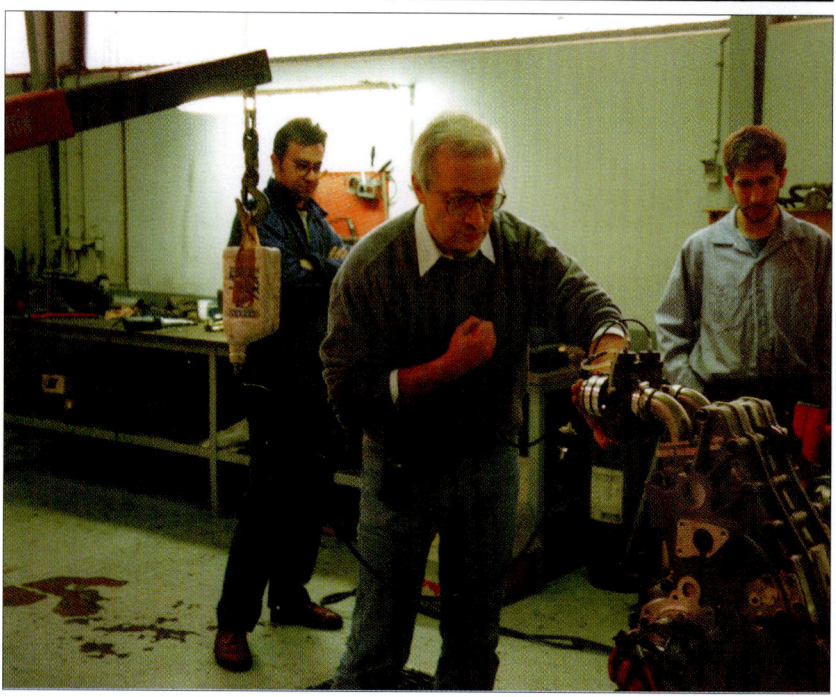

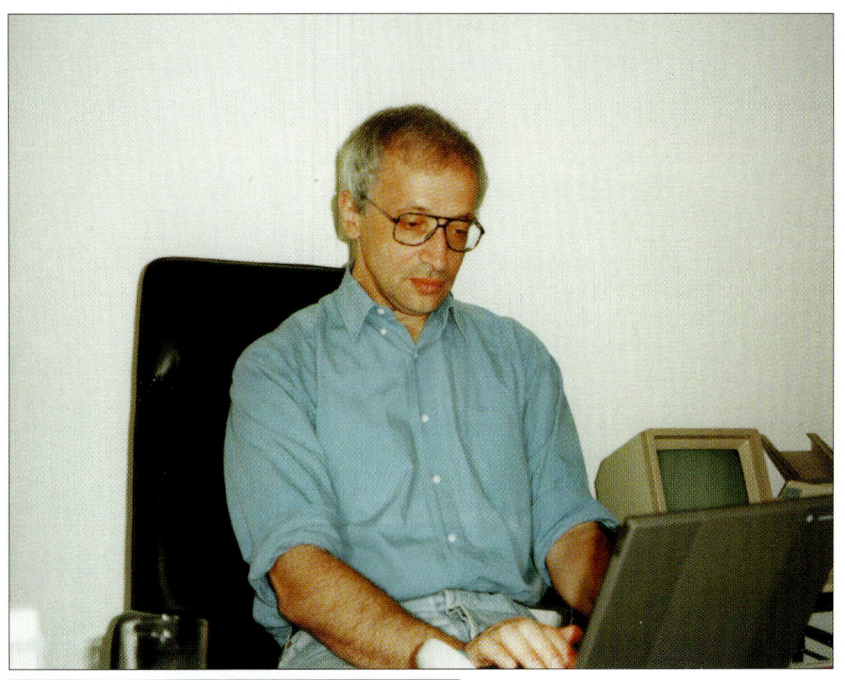

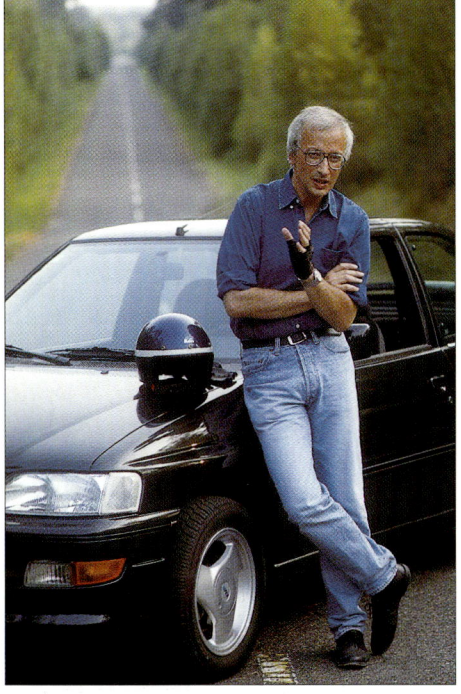

Writing My Story at home in Paris

At the Mortefontaine test track, near Paris

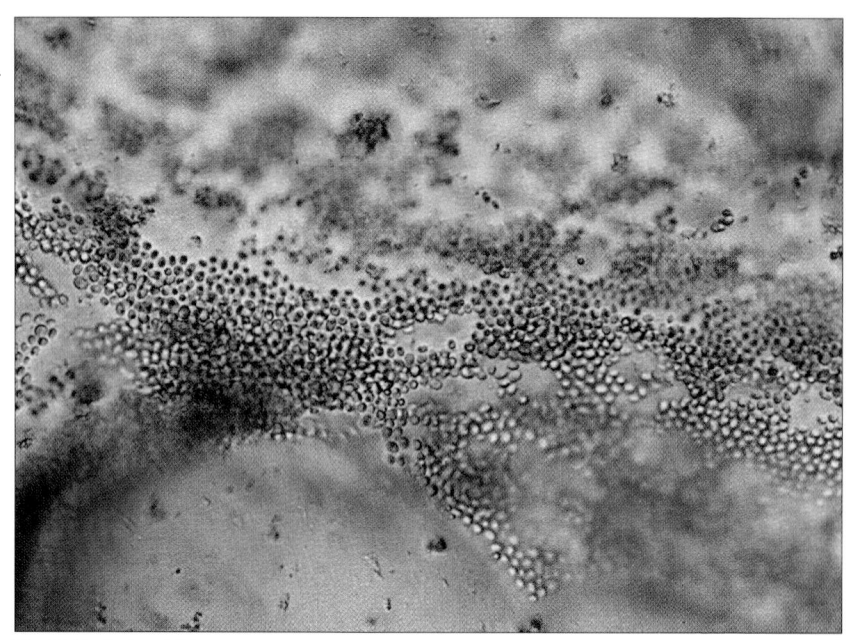

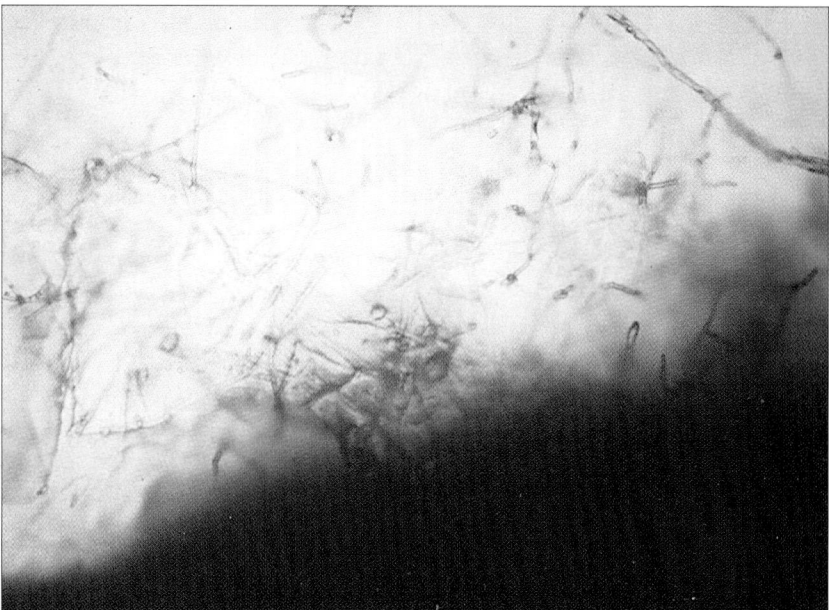

Microscopy photograph of fungal blastospores growing in nutrient medium around the plaques (top)

Microscopy photograph of fungal micellae growing from the plaque within the nutrient medium (below)

authorities if they were asked to explain why I was in a psychiatric clinic - although I doubted whether anybody would seriously enquire about me.

On that same evening I went to the psychiatric clinic accompanied by Tsvete and Shego who both had tears in their eyes. I explained the problem created by the intimidation of the state security agents to the lady doctor on duty.

On the following day the doctor went on holiday and a patient arrived whose sturdy, healthy appearance hardly suggested a treatable psychiatric condition. He announced his name as Kliment. From the very beginning the new patient kept a close eye on me and followed me wherever I went, even to the toilet. His main task was to see that I ate properly and in his efforts he even out-performed my grandmother. Kliment seemed to know everything about me. With a vacant expression he rummaged through all my belongings and dismantled my fountain-pen; probably looking for a micro-transmitter. It was not necessary for me to ask his profession because he hardly took the trouble to conceal that he was working for the Secret Service.

I could talk more openly to Kliment than had been the case with Sergey. Kliment hinted that the secret service considered my admission to the psychiatric hospital to be a brilliant defensive move. It was obvious that Mladenov's visit to Genscher had made some people nervous. Against that background our talks took an interesting turn. Kliment elaborated on two plans for the near future. In the first I would simply disappear. He quoted the example of a talented musician called Gencho who had vanished. The second plan, probably the suggestion of the heroes of the Quiet Front, implied the provision of a double who would substitute for me in all contacts with the West Germans. It was not clear what would happen to me in either of these two situations but it seemed logical to assume that I would be quietly liquidated.

Although I could not be sure that this was the case, I carelessly pointed out to Kliment that whatsoever plan was chosen for implementation, the West would be immediately informed. On the following day, my birthday, I was examined, declared healthy in body and mind and discharged from the clinic. Its manager, Doctor Dobrev, came to shake my hand and congratulated me on the publication abroad of my important work on medicine. The same day I read in the papers that Genscher had discussed bi-lateral cooperation while Mladenov had pointed out that to allow deployment of American middle-range missiles would undermine the détente.

I resumed my daily routine. On the surface nothing suggested that I had had a brush with state security. Telephoned threats ceased and I broke off all contacts with others save Tsvete, Bobby and Shego. I no longer talked even to Sergey and Tosho. I would take walks alone or sit drinking coffee by myself in the City Garden. Occasionally strangers would talk to me but I did not pursue any contact while I awaited the next round in the struggle. I anticipated that one day an article would be published abroad supporting my fungus research.

In mid-April I felt that I was being shadowed more intensively. Sergey and his team bumped into me too frequently in the street. What was happening? I felt intuitively that something must have been published abroad about my work.

At that time as an unusual sign of goodwill the authorities complied with certain provisions of the Helsinki Agreement by allowing selected Western newspapers to be sold in Sofia. At a newsstand I bought a copy of *Die Süddeutsche Zeitung* dated 19th April, only a couple of days after publication. Later that afternoon in my parents' flat Tsvete and I turned over its pages. Music coming from our small transistor radio was intended to jam any bugging devices in the room. On the second page Tsvete spotted a short article about a congress on internal diseases in Wiesbaden. As a student of German she was easily able to translate the title; *Medicine has not yet reached its full potential*.

The article ran for approximately twenty lines and told of about seven thousand hospital doctors from fifteen countries attending the congress organised to celebrate the centenary of the German Society for Internal Medicine. Hans Gotthard Lasch, a professor of coronary diseases from Giessen led the discussion on new aspects of the causes and treatment of heart attacks, immunotherapy, early diagnosis of cancer and stress management `more new discoveries, specific and effective therapies with reduced side-effects, the perfection of technique to help our patients' would be the answer to suggestions that medicine is approaching its effective limits, declared Lasch at the opening ceremony. No matter how carefully I studied the text, there seemed to be no hidden meaning. I was unable to deduce whether my research on the fungus had been discussed at the congress. Yet Professor Lasch's words left some room for interpretation, and in a strangely mysterious way I felt that my research would be discussed in Wiesbaden.

How might I have reached that conclusion? The very fact that I held in my hand a newspaper containing that piece of information was pure luck, just like seeing Teske at the Havana café the previous year. On the following day I searched for copies of other West German newspapers. I found articles on the Wiesbaden congress in *Die Frankfurter Allgemeine* of 19th April, in *Die Welt* of 20th April and again in *Die Süddeutsche Zeitung* of 21st April. But none of these articles contained the suggestion that my research had definitely been on the agenda.

While searching for newspapers I ran into agent Protogerov. We had little to say to each other but he was obviously eager to know whether I had any information on publication abroad of my work. At the same time the mysterious bearded customer of the Shapkite telephoned again to warn me that I would be in trouble if there was a campaign in my support abroad. I knew well the language of the secret service - this told me that there must have been some publication; most probably at Wiesbaden.

I visited Teske again at the West German embassy. I was told that he had left the country some time previously. In the following weeks nothing happened but I still felt that Wiesbaden was important to me. I then decided to discover who had represented Bulgaria at the congress. A pleasant young employee of the Ministry of Health told me that the central committee of the Party had sent two representatives to Wiesbaden; Prof. Nikolov, head of the Science Department of the Central Committee and Prof. Kaprelyan, rector of the Varna Medical Institute. She also told me that they had both submitted their reports to the Central Committee and not to the ministry as was the usual practice. In the end she asked me not to tell anyone that she had given me this information.

It seemed worthwhile to contact the professors for news. This would not be easy as the authorities were obviously determined to keep me in the dark. I decided that my chances of seeing Professor Nikolov were very slim but Professor Kaprelyan seemed more accessible. I told myself that I would have to act very cautiously if I wished to succeed in my approach.

At the beginning of July I took Viktor and Tsvete to the seaside for a holiday. We hired a tiny room in a cheap trade union holiday house in a resort fifteen minutes by bus from Varna. One morning instead of going to the beach I got on the bus to Varna and went to the medical institute. Varna's higher medical institute did not have a particularly academic air about it. In the dark corridor passing Professor Kaprelyan's room there was a long

Wiesbaden

line of students waiting for their faculty reports to be signed. They frowned at me as I walked past them right up to the door and knocked on it. A nervous secretary sitting at a desk loaded with papers asked what I wanted to which I replied that Roumen Antonov had arrived to see Professor Kaprelyan. I left the room.

It was a shot in the dark - if Professor Kaprelyan knew about me he would be willing to see me. If not all I could do was to take the bus back to the uncertainty of my present life.

A few minutes later the secretary opened the door and told me the professor was ready to see me.

I entered a large dark room. Professor Kaprelyan stood up behind his heavy desk to greet me. He was well into his fifties, a balding man with bushy black eyebrows. He said that he was very pleased to meet me personally and congratulated me on the very interesting research I had carried out. Then he asked me how I had discovered the idea of the fungus, where I worked and how I had carried out the joint research with the West German medical experts. I had to be very careful. It was a hot day. With my long hair, jeans and shirt I looked rather like a student. Professor Kaprelyan told me that he was surprised to see how young I looked despite being such an eminent researcher.

By avoiding all the difficult parts of my story I was able to answer his questions in a rather vague manner while trying to turn the conversation to the Wiesbaden congress. Kaprelyan said that he had learned about my theory and my experiments at the congress. Professor Lasch had presented experimental evidence confirming my theory of decomposing tissue. Kaprelyan pointed out that certain renowned names in world medicine at the congress had listened silently to the report without commenting. He thought that this was because they had been favourably impressed.

I asked Kaprelyan if he had any papers from the congress and he told me that all delegates had been given full documentation. He advised me that as head of the Bulgarian delegation Professor Nikolov would be better informed. He said that Nikolov had told him that my case had been considered by the Central Committee of the Party and I would probably now be sent to Western Germany. I had the feeling that although Kaprelyan obviously was unaware of the whole truth about me he seemed to be becoming naturally cautious.

I asked him if my research was of any interest to him and the Medical Institute. He said that after his return he had experimented on decomposing plaques taken from the aorta and the kidneys of a dead elderly woman and had observed the fungus for himself. He said that it looked horrible. Yet neither he nor his institute worked in that field and he was not an authority on the matter.

I had the feeling that Kaprelyan's spontaneous curiosity which had moved him to see me was beginning to wear thin and he was now feeling noticeably uncomfortable. The only thing left to me was to ask him once again whether he would allow me to see the congress documents about my research.

Kaprelyan agreed and said that he did not need them anyway. The papers were in a bag somewhere he said and looked in the drawers of his desk. After a while he decided that he must have left them at home and suggested that I call him the next day. I noted his phone number with the thought that something was troubling Kaprelyan. Perhaps he was already wondering whether it had been a good idea to see me after all. He suggested that I should contact pharmaceutical companies as they might be interested in my research. Once again he pointed out to me that he was no authority on the matter.

I left with the distinct feeling that Kaprelyan had become uneasy. Probably he would now call his party bosses to report on our meeting. I was not mistaken and when I called him the next day he told me that he was unable to find the congress papers. He never did, in fact. A few weeks later I realized that I would never get anything from him. I telephoned Professor Nikolov, the other delegate to the Wiesbaden congress, but he told me curtly that he could not remember which sessions he had attended.

This meant that the Iron Curtain had once again fallen into place.

Nevertheless my meeting with Kaprelyan proved that I had done something exceptional. By experimenting on myself since the end of 1979 under the most deplorable conditions, I had developed a ground-breaking theory in medicine. Despite my isolation and the increasing pressure of the Secret Service I had succeeded in surviving, sending my research abroad and eventually discovering that my work had been tested by specialists and finally presented to the world medical elite.

On reflection, I decided that after all I had done a good job. From my point of view, from now on it was only a matter of time before my fungus theory would be accepted. I felt very optimistic again and in my desperate isolation again fixed all my hopes on the elusive West.

In fact it was a few remarks let drop inadvertently by Kaprelyan that led me to speculate on what might have happened in Wiesbaden. Much of it remained unclear; I had not yet seen a single publication on the subject and what was the significance of the silence in which according to Kaprelyan the specialists at the congress had received my research? Could this mean that they found difficulty in understanding it, or were they rejecting it? Kaprelyan had been impressed by the silence but he could perhaps have been influenced by inside knowledge of my work and a feeling of inferiority in the presence of his Western colleagues. Still I told myself that as some of the finest specialists in the world had heard what Kaprelyan too had heard they surely would not ignore it. I rejected the possibility that my theory might remain unremarked without further investigation. It seemed to me that the world was not so absurd.

What did seem absurd however was the humiliating way in which the Bulgarian authorities continued to treat me. Nikolov had told Kaprelyan that the Party chiefs had discussed the possibility of sending me to the West. But Kaprelyan's cowardly behaviour after our meeting proved that the authorities would continue to regard me with suspicion. The initiators of the pressures applied to me had tried hard to conceal my research and keep my case in the dark. They showed no sign of letting me go and I was still under their firm control. There was not a single medical issue that could be more important to them than their constant struggle against capitalism. But what about West German interference? It seemed obvious that the diplomats had done all possible and the presentation of my research at the congress must mark the end of their efforts to help me. I could not imagine that West Germany would be prepared to jeopardize its relations with Bulgaria for my sake alone. In fact I wondered whether the presentation of my research to the public had not been done in accordance with conditions set by the Bulgarian authorities. It seemed at least that I was now recognized as the author of the theory but I decided that it was unlikely that I would learn anything about foreign research on it before the reports of the Wiesbaden congress were published.

I came to the conclusion that from now on my work would inevitably be recognized and all that I could do for the moment was to wait patiently, which of course was for me a familiar state. As always, whatever was happening appeared invisible to the others around me. I grew tired of trying to convince my relatives and friends about happenings which they could not see. I was unable to prove what I had heard from Kaprelyan and the methods of the secret service were also invisible. On the face of it I was an unemployed man fond of lonely walks. Perhaps some of my friends wondered whether I was in fact not in need of psychiatric help.

By the end of July my grandmother's health was deteriorating. She was as courageous as ever and made jokes about her approaching end. The last words she said to me were about her unwillingness to leave me before witnessing my success. At that she lost consciousness and after lying in a coma for two days died on 2nd August in my parents' flat. I still feel her loss deeply.

My father was rapidly losing weight. He refused to see the doctor but in September felt so ill that he had to be taken to hospital. The surgeon was no longer able to help and my father's cancer was obviously at an advanced stage. After the operation I stayed with him at the hospital and he asked me to say nothing to my mother and to spare her the news of his imminent death. I was at his bedside when he died on 14th October leaving me with a feeling of profound loneliness.

After that my life continued with as much difficulty as ever. Viktor and I moved back into my mother's flat. My sister had left after her marriage and I only had contact with Tsvete and occasionally with Bobby and Shego. They were both involved in love affairs and liked to discuss them over a glass of apple brandy at my home.

I was now into my second year of experimenting with 'M'. I still took the drug in small quantities and its effects continued in the familiar cycles. I concluded that the process could easily continue for another ten years and that I would be likely to undergo heavy curative crises, especially at the conclusion of some of the longer cycles.

All the time I kept searching for publications on what had happened at the Wiesbaden congress. I frequently visited the library of the Bulgarian Academy of Sciences and went through all reports and magazines in the hope that I might find a publication mentioning the 88th Wiesbaden Congress. At last at the end of the year the documentation from the congress arrived and Tsvete and I patiently traced every line and every page of the thick volumes. There was not a single word referring to the story Kaprelyan had told me.

That evening I sat in the kitchen with a cup of coffee thinking things over. There was only one possible conclusion to be drawn: the fungus theory and my experimental results had been presented at a closed session attended by Kaprelyan and this was why there was no publication.

I had experienced an absolutely unique opportunity to learn what had happened. Having read that short article in the newspaper I managed to trace one of the two men sent by the Communist Party to that same closed meeting in Wiesbaden. Furthermore the man in question had given me the information about what had happened simply because he had not yet been warned against it. But the items of information that I managed to obtain seemed very mysterious and only gave rise to more questions.

I had been absolutely certain that a publication about my research would appear. Following that logic I had gained access to Kaprelyan and his words had confirmed most of what I suspected might be going on since the time that Teske had accepted my work. Now I had to find out why the fungus theory and my experiments had been presented to a select group of eminent medical experts. The only things I had to go on was a few scraps of information and my methods of detection.

Though essentially simple, my fungus theory was profoundly revolutionary in the world of modern medicine. I was far more of an outsider in medicine than as a dissident opposing the regime in Sofia. However because I had been so preoccupied by resisting years of pressure from the State Security I had probably failed to appreciate how difficult it might be to launch my research abroad. I would give anything to learn about those who had worked on my theory but the only fact I had was that my articles had been handed over to the Max Planck Institute. Of course it would not be possible for these people to undermine the very foundations of modern medicine and replace them quickly. It would be necessary to find ways of making the theory and the experiment public and most probably that was why the theory had been presented discreetly to a select group of experts at a closed session of the congress.

Besides, I appreciated that medical research and new treatments in particular would not be publicised before the accumulation of sufficient supporting evidence. I was aware of publications in important medical magazines that had appeared only after long years of protracted research. I knew that I was unable to predict the outcome of the experiments on my own body. I could not even guess when the effects of 'M' would wear off and I certainly did not expect the press to publish articles that might lead to the public spontaneously deciding to self-administer 'M'.

Despite all these arguments there remained the fact that I had been kept completely in the dark about anything happening abroad that might be related to my work. It was now evident that the Bulgarian authorities had tried hard to suppress all information and prevent me from making contact with others. I could find no publication referring to my theory or to the articles that I had given Teske and I could not find my name mentioned anywhere. Was there a publication on my work after all or was I simply unable to locate it? Teske had promised to send me the answer of the Max Planck Institute but in fact I received nothing. The West German diplomatic service was discreet but could it be that its silence in my case was exaggerated? Could it be that the Bulgarian authorities had asked for that and had received a suitable undertaking?

Many more questions remained. Could some of the experts be interested in my idea and begin experiments after the closed session? What had happened to the research of the Max Planck Institute? Did Professor Lasch, the congress chairman, take part in that research? What about the Secret Service - would it continue to apply pressure on me?

I had no answers to these questions.

In the end I concluded that however mysterious things abroad might seem it was hardly possible that once begun, research on my theory would not be published. In any case I could do nothing better to launch my idea than what had been done at the Wiesbaden congress. I was now left with the belief that one day my theory would be publicly confirmed and then the Bulgarian authorities would no longer be able to keep me in the dark. Therefore I had to wait for a breakthrough in medicine in order to be able to leave the country. Emigration did not seem a quick and easy possibility. But at the end of 1982 I had no choice.

Wiesbaden

Neither did 1983 bring change. After the death of Brezhnev the system continued unchanged. A small inheritance left to us by grandmother and my father allowed mother, Viktor and me to live
modestly. My days passed uneventfully while I waited for something to happen. This period of calm seemed like a holiday after the recent stressful years. Sometimes I asked myself what would be the next chapter in my life. Anything was possible, varying from serious health problems arising from my continuing experimentation with 'M' to the publication of my research and great success. Tsvete grew restless about the future so I comforted her with the possibility that one day I might win a Nobel prize.

During the 89th congress in Wiesbaden nothing was mentioned about my research. Strangely I did not encounter any of the old familiar faces around Sergey although I could not believe that the secret service had forgotten entirely about me. Perhaps there too people were waiting for the results of my fungus experiment abroad and hoped that in the meantime I would remain forgotten and out of sight.

At the beginning of June the newspapers announced that in July Hans-Dietrich Genscher would again visit Bulgaria.

On 13th June I was summoned to appear before the district policeman, a young lieutenant with a surly expression. After questioning me about my activities he announced that I was not engaged in any activity of use to society and then asked me to sign a letter in which I undertook to find a job before the end of June. I was happy to oblige him.

Unemployment did not exist in the ideal socialist society of Bulgaria. The lieutenant explained to me that I could approach the manpower department of the district municipal office and that they would help me find a job. I went round to find that the only job available was for an unskilled worker in a food store. I took it. Then I wrote a letter to the police and handed it to the same district policeman. In my letter I pointed out to him that for over three years I had carried out a programme of medical research by experiment on myself. My research could perhaps be of some use to society but my work had been ignored and my appeals for cooperation left unanswered. Furthermore I insisted that I should be provided with information about the state of investigation of my theory in Bulgaria and abroad and I asked for cooperation in a further programme of experiment. At the end I warned that if I did not receive cooperation I would be forced to take a job as an unskilled worker. I considered this to be a severe disruption of my programme of scientific research and generally speaking to the disadvantage of Bulgaria.

The district policeman read my letter with steadily increasing irritation but nevertheless agreed to accept it.

Despite all this, on 20th June I took a job as an unskilled worker in a food store with the task of unloading trucks and stacking the goods in the warehouse.

Chapter Thirteen
The Price of Freedom

As I unloaded crates of cooking oil, barrels of feta and boxes of food I no longer expected that my destiny could be influenced by events such as Genscher's forthcoming visit. Genscher came to Sofia on 14th July and departed on the following day. The newspapers briefly referred to his dissatisfaction with the progress of scientific and technical cooperation between West Germany and Bulgaria while his Bulgarian counterpart Mladenov was rumoured to have observed that middle-range missiles remained an obstacle to a congenial political climate in Europe.

I did not find his visit exciting, however. Work in the food store was hard but at least I seemed to have been abandoned by the agents of State Security. This fact together with the pleasant weather made my life more bearable. There was no point in discussing my personal problems with the two guys working with me in the warehouse.

A very pretty nineteen year-old girl worked as a cashier. Once as we were standing next to the bottles of whisky and vodka I told her that I preferred whisky. At the end of the day the young cashier asked me in a mysterious voice to follow her into the warehouse. There she opened a bottle of whisky and I felt my guardian angels sent to protect me from seduction were having a hard time for although I was approaching forty I still seemed attractive to women. On this occasion I did not give in but it cost me nearly as much effort as in unloading the vans. This girl was extremely beautiful, had a sense of humour and claimed that she was in love with me. The inner struggle of resisting her advances became a daily trial.

Tsvete was getting nervous about me and the future. Her enthusiasm of the past years was vanishing with the passing of time and she insisted that I should find my correct place in society and cease to be an outsider. She no longer believed in me and we argued constantly.

I patiently waited for the day when my fungus research would be published. As I continued to take satisfaction in inventing things I began to think about a four-stroke engine with a simpler construction than the one that I had earlier patented. This brought back the pleasant evening hours when I pored over a piece of paper and made sketches. Could I find a better solution than my earlier invention? I decided that this time I would keep my work secret until I left the country.

I had taken 'M' for four consecutive years. By the end of 1983 I decided to stop taking the drug to see whether my body had developed immunity to the fungus and whether the process of curative crises would continue without the medicine as I had observed in the case of my younger volunteers. It transpired that I was now immune to the fungus and the process continued.

That was an interesting result but I realized that I could not put an end to that process even if I wanted to and I wondered whether I should expect some heavy crises in coming years.

At the beginning of 1984 I found a new job as an assistant art director in a TV movie. At the time one of West Germany's most wanted terrorists had been sighted in a Bulgarian holiday resort.

Commissioned by the secret service, the TV movie had to convince viewers that the CIA supported these terrorists with the aim of discrediting the Bulgarian authorities. My career in the movie business was strange to say the least; ten years ago I had been the art director of a movie about a scientist who discovered an anti-cancer drug and was then exposed as a traitor and a villain working for a Western intelligence service. What did the scriptwriters of the secret service think of my story so far?

The team went to a small town near the Greek border to shoot a couple of scenes but I was not allowed to go with them. The police refused to allow me to visit the border region so I resigned and took up yet another job as an art teacher.

Time passed by. I still expected that a publication on my fungus research would appear but nothing suggested that it was imminent. In any case, the secret service seemed to have lost interest in me and I was quite unaware of its presence, even if I were still under surveillance.

Taking advantage of that relatively quiet period, I decided to apply for a permit to leave for West Germany. I was now forty and could no longer expect to begin a new career. Moreover no-one in the country seemed to take the slightest interest in my medical research. Again I sought logic; what was the point of preventing me from going abroad if outside my country at least I could carry out useful research to help sick people?

With that argument in mind I applied for a permit from the passport department quoting the events at the Wiesbaden Congress in 1981. After the automatic refusal I insisted on seeing the head of the department and explained to him how important my work could be. The chief said that if I continued to harass him he would ask for an investigation into how and why I had sent my work abroad.

I therefore tried again and sent a letter to the Minister of the Interior. There was no answer.

Finally I wrote to Zhivkov asking to be allowed to leave the country to pursue my medical research. I addressed the letter to the State Council. Again there was no answer. I went to the information desk and an ugly employee assured me that the State Council could be of no assistance to me.

To get a clear idea of exactly where I stood, I filed for a permit to go to Czechoslovakia. That should not have been a problem as anybody was allowed to travel to Czechoslovakia. It transpired that anyone did not include me. I knew no one who had been refused permission to visit another communist country.

Thus after seventeen attempts to go abroad I was forced to conclude that I was now doomed to stay in Bulgaria for ever.

In 1984 the ancient Chernenko came to power in the Soviet Union and with demented and dogmatic conformity intensified confrontation with the West. In Bulgaria communists went about saying that a possible military conflict might not be that bad after all. It could even make things better. In that bleak period

Genscher again visited Sofia in March 1985 but a day later Chernenko died having failed to start a new world war.

In reflecting on that situation I concluded that Genscher was more interested in developing good relations with Bulgaria than in insignificant problems like mine. Possibly my case was no longer on his agenda at all. In the following years Genscher again visited Bulgaria a couple of times - in 1986 in the Gorbachev era and then again in 1987 as Chancellor of West Germany. He came again in 1990 as a consultant to the former communist government of Mladenov. After all that it seemed that Genscher must have got along fairly well with Mladenov during those years.

In 1985 I discovered a new four-stroke engine solution. My new design was simpler and easier to make than the one covered by my earlier patent. I made a scale model of it using Meccano and cardboard and often toyed with it in the search for potential disadvantages or a better solution, but the present one seemed to be the best under all circumstances. As I write these lines an exact metal replica of the scale model has been made and is functioning perfectly. At the time I kept my work secret, waiting for the day when I would leave Bulgaria.

One day I ran into Rusi Dundakov, a fellow student from the Academy of Fine Arts. Ten years had passed since I had left the Cinema Centre and the Fine Artists Union in whose club I used to meet Rusi. I told him about my experiment and the fungus research. Rusi always defied common logic and took spontaneous, intuitive decisions. This time he decided to offer his services as a volunteer and follower of my theory. I was very pleased to see him, and after long years of enforced isolation I enjoyed the company of an old friend and a unique sense of humour. We took to meeting in the studio café of Ekran (screen) a TV company where Rusi worked as an art director.

He offered me a job as assistant art director for a children's movie. My task was to make a strange-looking car that flew and obeyed orders. After long discussions about its construction we decided to fix a couple of boxes on a chassis with open wheels. Thus I designed the first car to be made for the film. I did not like it but had to be practical. I found a mechanic and together we built a car out of bits from an old Zaporozhets, pieces of pipe and panels of wood. Hidden away in a red box, the engine quickly overheated and the car could only be driven for ten minutes at a time. The tricky part was that I was supposed to drive the car myself hidden away in the black box with only a tiny slit through which I could hardly see a thing. The TV crew went to shoot at the seaside and I felt that my life was not at all difficult. I patiently waited for news on fungus research and kept wondering what might have happened to it.

Time went by. In 1986 I decided that four years after the Wiesbaden congress the silence was deafening. What did the people at the Max Planck Institute do? Was there a publication?

Why did no-one write to me or seek contact with me? Could it be that someone had tried to but had failed to penetrate the wall built around me? Those questions were constantly disturbing.

I decided to write a letter to Professor Lasch. As chairman of the Wiesbaden congress of 1982 he must have been in touch with events. I described what I had heard from Kaprelyan and asked Lasch to do everything possible to get in touch with me, suggesting a possible visit to Sofia. My experimentation was now in its seventh year and the various curative crises continued although in the last four years I had taken no more 'M'. I believed that my observations were of importance to the continuing fungus research. I wrote the letter in Bulgarian and gave copies to several people who left for abroad asking them to post it. At least one of the letters must have reached Professor Lasch at his university clinic in Giessen, yet I never received an answer.

After having tried so hard to discover what had happened I decided finally that it was time to adopt a different strategy for leaving the country since I could no longer rely on my expectations that the fungus research might be published.

I was alone. Tsvete had finally abandoned her love for me; as I returned from a few days spent on the film set she did not come to see me. She could no longer stand the situation and there was nothing I could do to make her change her mind.

Gorbachev had launched perestroika, but very little of its influence could be felt in Sofia. The regime showed no signs of abandoning its grip on affairs. People like me could never hope to leave the country.

There was one single possibility to escape that I had not yet tried. Ten years after the Helsinki Agreement which included provisions for marriages between citizens of different nationalities, to marry a foreigner was the last, perhaps humiliating, opportunity of legally leaving the country for those who had no other hope. It was still necessary for the authorities to give their permission for marriage to a foreigner and I assumed that it would not be easy for me; Colonel Uzunov having declared that I would not be granted permission to marry if I applied. I remembered that Lyubo Kanov had left Bulgaria after marrying a Canadian.

In recent years I had resisted the advances of many women. Rusi thought that that was a sin especially when beautiful women were concerned. I felt the weight of the twenty years since my first attempt to leave Bulgaria and it seemed irrelevant to resist temptation any more. I seemed to be faced with one final choice: either marry a foreigner or spend my old age in the country of my birth. Thus I decided to find a suitable wife. I never imagined that there could be a chapter about this in my future book and I hardly felt ready for it. My lonely research on the fungus had been arduous and its launch rather like an adventure movie. After all that had happened there seemed to be only one possible role for me and this had very little to do with intellectual activity.

I had no West European women friends and had to wait for a chance meeting to occur. While walking one day on the Ruski Boulevard a French woman with short brown hair asked me about the Nevski cathedral. We began a conversation and I asked her to have coffee with me, which is how I met Anne, a Parisienne on holiday in Bulgaria. I decided to be frank with her and told her hnow important a marriage was to me. Anne was aged about thirty, an energetic, sociable woman who did not look like someone about to marry a stranger chatting to her in a Sofia street. Nevertheless she gave me her address and soon wrote to me.

I wrote back and proposed to her again. I had already married twice for love and was hardly in a position to say that I expected to be happy with a woman whom I barely knew. The only argument I was able to put forward was my willingness to take a chance if she would agree to do the same. Anne seemed reserved but invited me to visit her in Paris. I telephoned her to ask whether she liked cooking and then thanked her for the invitation with the reminder that I was not allowed

The Price of Freedom

to leave the country. I invited her to come and visit me again, but she was not ready to return to Sofia and joked about it. I told myself that I must find another foreigner.

At the end of 1987 Anne wrote to me after a long period of silence saying that she was ready to come to Sofia to discuss the possibility of marriage. This time it was too late because I was about to marry another Parisienne who in fact had already accepted my proposal.

During 1986 I was working on a movie in which the youthful producer Nikolay Akimov recounted his childhood memories. He was a short young man with a short black beard and an indecisive and ambitious but kind personality. My friend Rusi was his art director and Akimov was under the influence of Rusi and me to the extent that we were soon able to suggest the inclusion of events and personalities into the movie.

One day at the café of the Ekran studio a beautiful woman with short blonde hair and a mini-skirt sat at the table next to ours. She made a deep impression on us and Rusi and I ceased discussion of our work on the movie as we sat there drinking coffee. Rusi still invented stories in which female attraction was the main topic. He made a few remarks about the strange blonde woman and Akimov then asked her to come for a screen test as a result of which she was offered the main role in the movie which she accepted. That is how I met the Russian Larisa. She was not a professional actress but just happened to be married to an obscure and miserable-looking movie producer.

The film was to be shot in Troyan, a small town in the Balkan mountains where Akimov had been born. There was no hope that I might meet a foreigner there and I accepted the mission as just another setback to my plans for emigration. The atmosphere was easy-going; no-one worked at all and I realized that Larisa was making extraordinarily energetic advances towards me. She was a short blonde with sparkling blue eyes who accompanied herself on the guitar as she sang romantic Russian songs that she had composed herself.

For quite a while I resisted her blandishments in my attempt to convince Larisa that her attempts at seduction were futile since I had already proposed to Anne. Larisa was not willing to abandon the chase and refused to hide her love although she was already married with a child.

As I gave in to the temptation I told myself that our romance would end when we left Troyan.

At that time I visited Vanga the clairvoyant who had invited me to consult her via Uzunov's daughter some years earlier. A fellow artist arranged for a permit to take me in his Trabant to her little house. As we pulled up, a man came out of the house, walked up to us and called out my name. It was a strange experience, for no-one knew that I was coming and there were a hundred or so people outside waiting to be received.

Vanga was an old blind woman. Her closed eyes gave her face a tranquil expression. Before I could say anything she asked about the medicine that I had used and how I had applied it. Then she announced that I had been cured from cancer of the jaw. Her telepathic abilities were amazing and her way of expressing herself very simple. She inquired about my therapy and then said that it was my turn to ask questions of her. I was eager to know when I would be able to leave the country. She interrupted me and said that I had to get married first. I asked her about my future work and the fungus research and she told me that I would make more successful inventions and that my rights to the fungus theory would one day be recognized but that it would take time and by then the scandal surrounding my work would become public knowledge.

Vanga's gift of clairvoyance was impressive. Reflecting on her words I realized that I had only one choice and that was definitely to marry a foreigner.

Regrettably my romance with Larisa did not come to an end at the conclusion of the movie shoot. I tried to explain to her how doomed was our love affair; she was married and I was seeking a wife. However she ignored my words and swore that she loved me with all her heart.

In the evenings I sat with a sheet of paper testing my inventive ability. Once again I developed my old idea for an automatic gearbox and a limited-slip differential. At those times I told myself that Larisa's love had no place in my totally disrupted life, but despite my resistance, her boundless energy and love prevailed.

By the end of the year Larisa had divorced her husband. Born and bred in Dnepropetrovsk in a system far more rigid than the Bulgarian copy, she was an emotionally reckless, strong-minded intelligent woman. Her feelings dominated her life and she was prepared to sacrifice all for their sake. She had no self-pity and joked lightly about her emotional life.

In the summer of 1987 a group of friends put me in touch with Edith. She was willing to come to Sofia to discuss marriage. I told Larisa about Edith and she agreed that to marry her was my best course. Larisa was very brave in her disappointment and at our parting she told me that no-one could ever love me as much as she did. I must admit that my time with Larisa was very happy.

Edith arrived in September. She was a short Parisienne with big brown eyes and blonde hair. When Bobby and I went to meet her she seemed sad and pensive. Bobby came to help as interpreter. It was not going to be easy to bridge the gap between us before we would be ready to decide to live together. Edith was a modest woman without illusions. As a divorcée she did not expect life to be easy and the reason for coming all the way from Paris was that she too was looking for a partner in marriage. Edith had consulted a clairvoyant before leaving for Sofia and had been told that we would marry. She already had doubts about our relationship and was jealous and insecure.

I applied for a permit to marry. The period within which an answer should be expected passed and I felt uneasy. Finally after an extended delay at the end of the year I was authorised to marry Edith. The first available date at the municipal registry office was 21st January, my forty-fourth birthday, and that was when I married Edith who thus became my third wife.

This event meant that after seventeen unsuccessful attempts during the last twenty years I was now finally in a position to leave Bulgaria. I simply could not believe that my efforts to escape that had begun by climbing the hills near Trieste in the autumn of 1967 had now come to an end. I felt that I had paid a heavy price to gain my freedom by wasting all those years. Yet I had decided that there was no reason why I should be disappointed; there were many who would give far more than I to be in my position. For me freedom came rather late in life, but still it came.

The Price of Freedom

I applied for a passport and was given one in February. The French visa was issued in April and I immediately booked a flight to Paris on 29th of that month.

All my friends, Bobby, Shego, and Rusi came to see me off. Mother cried with joy. Viktor expected to receive his passport within a few months and to join me in Paris. He was still under age and legally in my custody.

That day the weather in Sofia was gloomy. On the way to the airport I suffered from stomachache since at that time I was going through a heavy curative crisis. I peered at the streets through which I had taken so many lonely walks, wondering when I would see them again. On the Ruski Boulevard the taxi stopped to allow a disabled man to slowly cross the street and I wondered what would happen to my fellow citizens left behind in the tender care of the regime.

The plane took off but I was not excited. I felt as though I was in a strange dream. The two hours of the flight passed quickly and then I saw Paris from the window. The weather was sunny and I could clearly see the Eiffel Tower.

I knew that I had to make a new start in life but had no idea how.

Chapter Fourteen
The Antonov Automatic Gearbox

As I arrived in Paris during the sunny afternoon of 29th April 1988, everything around me seemed amazing and of another world. During the evening I sat alone in a café in the Place d'Italie reflecting on how I should begin my new life.

Here I was at last, free at the age of forty-four. In my pocket I had the 150 francs allowed by the Bulgarian authorities - just sufficient for fifteen cups of coffee. My English was poor and my French even worse. The only people I knew in this bewildering city were my wife and a Bulgarian with whom I expected to sign a contract to exploit my inventions.

For more than eight years I had experimented with a drug that had given me the evidence I needed to substantiate my fungus theory and this activity had become the most important thing in my life. I knew that I had to complete the task begun in 1980 and make my research public knowledge. For the first time in my life I was free to contact whomever I wished in the world and more than that I was now extremely eager to discover what had happened after Teske had accepted my papers in 1981.

On 9th May 1988 I visited the West German embassy in Paris and spoke to the Cultural Attaché, Werner Burkart. I told him about Teske and the information Kaprelyan had provided and asked him to make inquiries for me. Burkart promised to do so and to contact me.

During the last eight years I had failed in my endeavours to make my fungus research public knowledge and did not imagine that this time I would be in a position to make a medical breakthrough. It seemed easier to me to try to interest the motor industry in one of my inventions although such an enterprise seemed anything but simple to me. Of all my inventions the four-stroke engine from 1985 was in the most advanced stage, but it would take a great deal of money and time to introduce a new engine and in my position I had neither.

During recent years I had also worked on the design of an automatic gearbox. My mechanical models were not as accurate as those that I had made for the four-stroke engine but I had had a couple of ideas that promised simpler solutions to those available with existing automatic gearboxes. The present family of automatic gearboxes invented in the States during the 1940s was outdated and inefficient. European cars were generally smaller and fitted with manual gearboxes. Automatic transmissions were accepted as more expensive, more thirsty, offering reduced acceleration and speed while being heavier and larger than the manual equivalent. It seemed to me that a more efficient automatic gearbox would attract considerable interest and I believed that with modest investment I would be able to build and install an automatic gearbox in a car to demonstrate its advantages over existing ones. This was an optimistic idea that at the time seemed to me the best way to make a fresh start.

On the day following my arrival I began negotiations for capital investment in my automatic gearbox project. Michail Avramov, the only Bulgarian I knew in Paris, had arrived a year earlier. He was aware of my work and willing to help me negotiate with a private French investor to whom he was related. Michail was a soft, polite man interested in finance and later founded an investment company himself. At the time however, he was taking his first steps and drew up an investment contract for my invention. I agreed to pay him ten per cent of the profits from the patent that I had just filed in France in exchange for one hundred thousand francs to be paid in a year. During that period the invention had to be demonstrably successful and if not the investor could take over my rights to the patent. Nevertheless I succeeded in including a contractual clause stipulating that in the case of failure I had the choice to concede my rights only on one of three patents offered as security of which one only related to the automatic gearbox.

The money I received amounted to the equivalent of a year's unemployment benefit. I decided to construct a small prototype of the automatic gearbox and to install it in radio-controlled model car with a 5cc glowplug engine. Using miniature parts I built a car producing a deafening noise. It was not easy to operate it and at its very high speeds it constantly bumped into objects around it. All there was now to do was to introduce my idea to the motor industry.

Hoping to attract interest in the excellent capacity for acceleration of the small car, I approached a couple of French companies with the offer to demonstrate my model to them. My prototype had already been tested by a model car racing driver who had reached the conclusion that my automatic gearbox gave far better acceleration than that of standard, single-speed models. An engineer from one of the companies contacted agreed to attend my demonstration and as we met he told me that he had seen hundreds of inventions of which none had even passed the point of demonstration. Yet he operated my model car until the fuel tank was empty and seemed to be impressed. In the end he said it would take time to consider the idea and warned me not to expect a quick answer.

As I waited for answers from Burkart, the West German Cultural Attaché, and the car company engineer I began to adapt to my new life. I was quick to realize that this was going to be difficult. Before emigrating I had lived in isolation but that was nothing compared to my present situation.

Unable to speak French and with few contacts I felt helpless and lost in Paris. My Bulgarian nationality did not provide an easy start in the world and besides I had very little time in which to adapt.

Edith supported me in a calculated manner and never exceeded the limits that she had laid down. She was unwilling to tolerate me fiddling with parts and building my prototype in her kitchen and so to avoid an unpleasant scene I rented a small flat near the Pont de Tolbiac with a miserable view of railway lines and old houses near the Seine. I lived there alone; Edith did not visit me and remained in her own house.

At my address in Paris I never received any good news. The Bulgarian authorities refused to allow my son Viktor to join me although he was under age and still in my custody. The head of the passport department behaved arrogantly when my son went to see him and I did not expect that he would ever succeed on obtaining a passport - all I could do was to continue to seek support in Paris.

The engineer who had attended the demonstration of my gearbox had not yet answered. No other car companies seemed interested in my invention despite my approaches. Burkart had failed to contact me since our meeting so three months later on 9th August 1988 I sent him a letter repeating my questions about Teske and Kaprelyan. His answer came on 19th August. Burkart told me that inquiries made on behalf of the embassy at the Max Planck Institute, the German Society for Internal Medicine, Professor Lasch and the West German embassy in Sofia had led to what he called `negative results'.

For a long time I stared at the letter trying to make something of it.

The West German authorities had remained silent about all events from my first meeting with Teske up to the Wiesbaden congress and the news given to me by Kaprelyan. None of the delegates attending the closed session had accepted my idea or had been interested to follow it up. Probably the silent rejection of my theory had discouraged those who had given it their initial support and the diplomats had probably put away all documents into their secret files. Could it have been the Bulgarian authorities who had insisted on that course? It was a fact that Genscher and Mladenov had a close and friendly relationship.

I was appalled - was there anything remaining from my efforts to publish my research in 1981? It was obvious that there had never been any publication and when I made enquiries of the Library of Congress in Washington and discovered a summary of my article on physics there was nothing to be traced on the subject of my fungus theory.

I stared out of the window at the Seine and contemplated the difficult task ahead of me. What could I do after all this time to make my research public? It seemed to me that I was now in a worse position to undertake anything than at any time in the recent past.

I went out for a long walk in that deserted neighbourhood that is one of the gloomiest in Paris. It was a sunny day however and gradually I marshalled my thoughts and concluded that although absurd, the world was *comme ça*. If there was anything that I could do at the moment it would be to continue with my efforts to launch the automatic gearbox. If that brought me success I might be able to make my fungus research public. This was a desperate strategy but it seemed I had to make one miracle occur if I wanted to witness a second. However anything would be better than to abandon all that I had done so far. This made me determined to succeed with the automatic gearbox.

I could base my hopes only on the opinion of one engineer who although he had not yet accepted my invention, had not yet rejected it. His hesitation might be just sufficient encouragement to persuade me to continue with the automatic gearbox. Even if his eventual reaction to my invention was favourable that would only give a boost to the project and would not provide me with employment or income. The automatic gearbox could only be allowed to demonstrate its advantages over existing types if it could be installed in a car and this was something I could not yet afford.

Both the time and the money from the first investment contract were slipping away. I had to look for new contracts and opportunities before I ran out of funds. Edith was reluctant to share the risks of my gearbox enterprise.

I searched my memory for people I knew who might be in Paris. There were a few of them and I found the telephone number of a former classmate who had defected twenty years before. I telephoned him and we arranged to meet. He introduced me to people in his circle.

By the end of the year I moved out of my flat near the Pont de Tolbiac. Edith and I had gradually drifted apart and it was obvious that our marriage was a failure. We divorced in the following year.

At that time I had one of my rare strokes of good fortune: I met Roxanne, a tall, energetic and logical American with red hair and dark blue eyes. She worked in Paris and knew a lot of people. To her the world was the right place to do things and she offered to help me in any way possible.

The Bulgarian authorities continued to refuse to allow my son Viktor to join me. I wrote to the French Foreign Ministry and to the Red Cross asking them to help him but there was little result beyond some spiteful remarks from the Bulgarian consul in Paris. By the end of the year it was announced that President Mitterrand would visit Sofia. The French press criticised the planned visit by pointing out the reluctance of the Bulgarian communist regime to relinquish its grip on society. On 20th December I wrote to Mitterrand asking him to intercede with the Bulgarian authorities on behalf of my son and took the letter to the presidential office. In January, on my forty-fifth birthday, Mitterrand visited Sofia. Would my request have any effect?

A few days later, Viktor now aged sixteen, was given permission to leave the country and I met him in Paris at the beginning of May.

In the meantime the engineer who had agreed to examine my gearbox ran various computer models on its performance and achieved positive results. By the end of 1988 he even seemed enthusiastic about the idea but his company was not interested. That was the beginning of the adventurous launch of the Antonov automatic gearbox. Today, ten years later, it would take a book to describe the whole story. Maybe I will attempt to write that one day, but it is not easy to describe all the ups and downs in a nutshell.

To begin with, I had run out of money. That year I was supposed to apply for a world patent on the gearbox that would cost at least twice as much as the initial investment. I tried to attract the interest of my investor but we failed to reach agreement and he decided against any further funding of the gearbox.

I then applied for a subsidy from the French governmental organisation ANVAR, which specialised in the promotion of inventions. ANVAR examined patent applications and assisted with patent protection with a maximum financial subsidy of one hundred and fifty thousand francs. I was fortunate to receive the maximum subsidy and reflected bitterly on my financial adventures as an inventor.

Roxanne offered me a small investment too and with it I decided to build a prototype of the gearbox to use in a kart. The engineer sent me some parts of automatic gearboxes manufactured by his company, to help.

I found a mechanic, a former motorcycle racer who repaired bikes in a tiny dusty workshop in Yvry. While waiting for clients he would spend his days drinking beer, an activity he was reluctant to abandon even when he did get a job. Together we began to build my automatic gearbox in an old kart. Finally after much work the kart ran in the small workshop yard. Roxanne invited some friends and we demonstrated the prototype with success; one of her friends, a retired company director, was interested to invest in my invention.

This was the beginning of the next stage. I signed a contract with my new investor. The goal was to install a full-sized prototype of the gearbox in a car. I bought an old Peugeot 305 long past its best and from a nearby junkyard, an automatic gearbox. The junkyard was in a housing estate to the south of Paris among small ugly houses with broken fences. I heaved the heavy gearbox into the boot of the car and paused for a rest. With my greasy hands I lit a cigarette and thought of the long road ahead from the Yvry junkyard to the glamorous car industry.

With my decrepit Peugeot and the old gearbox which I intended to dismantle for parts I began my struggle with the highly advanced technology of the automatic gearbox. Even in his moments of sobriety the Yvry mechanic hardly fancied my chances. Would I succeed? I was convinced that I would.

The Antonov Automatic Gearbox 149

There was very little that I could do to promote my fungus research. Roxanne supported my theory and had contacted a couple of physicians in France and the USA but none was willing to repeat my experiment. She did not abandon hope and one day came to me with good news; she had managed to track the telephone number and address of Rudolf Teske in Düsseldorf. In the evening we telephoned him. Teske sounded surprised and asked how I had obtained his telephone number. He said that he remembered our meetings but seemed reluctant to discuss them. He could not remember to whom he had passed the materials that I had given him in 1981.

A few days later, on 7th March 1989, I wrote to him about the information given to me by Professor Kaprelyan on his return from the Wiesbaden congress in 1982. To this I added a copy of the article I had given him in 1981 and a copy of Burkart's letter from the West German embassy in Paris. I also sent a copy of the same letter to Professor Lasch. Lasch did not reply but Teske replied three months later with a letter dated 2nd July.

He had sent my letter and copies of the documentation to a friend of his, the president of the World Association of Medical Historians, Professor Schadewaldt from Düsseldorf University. Professor Schadewaldt had found no publication concerned with my research. Teske hoped that the professor, a pathologist, would express an opinion on my research, but I never heard anything from him.

Teske ended his letter with the words 'the papers you gave me in Sofia were sent to the Max Planck Institute but I regret to say that I really do not remember having received a reply and it is quite possible that this did not reach me, as I left Sofia in 1982'.

That letter is the only written evidence of what might have happened to my fungus research so far. I told myself that one day I would learn more about it and because everything depended on how successful the automatic gearbox would be, I persisted in my work.

I concentrated on my first prototype in the dusty Yvry workshop, which even lacked facilities to install the gearbox in the car. There were few tools and the mechanic filed the few pieces of metal that would not fit when we tried to assemble them. Nevertheless one day the gearbox was ready and we went to a garage where we could install it in the Peugeot. The mechanic knew the owner who gave us three hours to work on the car. The last pieces were assembled in the street outside. At last I sat behind the wheel and started the engine.

Despite everything the Peugeot burst into life and I drove with surprise and excitement through the small streets of the neighbourhood. My automatic gearbox prototype however was in bad shape. The primitively adapted parts jammed on the following day and I stood helplessly by the old Peugeot that had come to a halt just outside Paris; stubbornly refusing to start.

What could I do with my bare hands to get that car to run again? My battle with advanced automatic gearboxes was going to be a long and arduous struggle.

We removed the gearbox in the garage and I took it to the small studio near the Arc de Triomphe where Viktor and I now lived. He helped me drag the gearbox to the tiny bathroom where I dismantled it. The various parts had damaged each other and the bathroom became covered in filthy oil full of metal particles. I refused to give in to despair and after vainly trying to clean my filthy hands, went to bed.

I later managed to reassemble the gearbox and install it in the car after making some improvements but I was not yet ready to trust it and made no more demonstrations.

I had begun discussions with an organisation called APELOR. Because the state-owned French coalmines were so inefficient, APELOR provided assistance in training miners for other work and was also prepared to subsidise companies able to provide employment in mining districts.   Within its programme APELOR allocated financial resources to promote inventions; the subsidy being provided not in the form of money but in services offered by the mining workshops in Lorraine.   APELOR agreed to consider a project to install a prototype of my automatic gearbox in a car at its expense.

Four engineers from the Lorraine mines came to Paris to drive the Peugeot.   They were all somewhat overweight so I was prepared for a breakdown at any time while driving through the Paris streets.   Fortunately everything went well and only as I was parking the car did the gearbox jam, which they fortunately failed to notice.   All of them left, duly impressed.

One day while driving through Paris I heard the news of the fall of the Berlin Wall on the car radio.   For a moment I could not believe it.   I parked the car and entered the first café I saw. Yes it was true but the people around me did not seem to understand the full implications of this momentous happening.   The world had certainly changed but no-one seemed to care although I felt like shouting with excitement.   A beggar asked me for money and I gave him everything I had in my pocket, much to his surprise.   I drank a whisky and took a long walk.   I stayed up the whole night watching enthusiastic Berliners on the TV.   These events seemed so improbable but the fall of communism spread like wildfire to all East European countries and by the end of the year I saw thousands of my fellow countrymen thronging the streets of Sofia.   I felt an overwhelming urge to return to Bulgaria to join the cheering, singing crowds, and then I realized that for me it was rather late.   The only thing I could do for the future of my country was to make a success of my work.

At the beginning of 1990 I signed a contract with APELOR and the Lorraine mines to develop my automatic gearbox and install it in a car.   The value of the subsidy in the form of labour and workshop time amounted to seven hundred and fifty thousand francs.   My obligation was to stay with my company in Lorraine if the project was successful.   This subsidy at last gave my invention a real chance of success and I asked myself how it could have been allocated to me.   Later I dined with a former French diplomat who had worked in Sofia and who told me that the French authorities knew about my visits to the West German embassy and that it was my reputation that had secured the subsidy.   At last the risks that I had taken in the past appeared to have paid off.   As an immigrant I had been given this unique opportunity and I was determined to make a success of it.

In February I went to Lorraine to work on the prototype, settling in Merlebach, a small mining town near the German border.   This was the middle of Europe and yet somehow it seemed very remote and quiet; perhaps because already several mines in the district had been closed.   Merlebach was one of the peaceful towns near Forbach where France ends and Germany begins.   The local people were very calm by nature and spoke French with a heavy accent; the elderly among them in fact spoke a German dialect.   A few miles across the border lay Saarbrucken with its beautiful hills and bridges over the River Saar that was where the leading German company ZF had its automatic gearbox factory.

I now changed my concept of the automatic gearbox.   The new one operated on a different principle; the original incorporating one type of stepless gear-change system. The prototypes built for the radio-controlled model car, the kart and the Peugeot were based on that principle which I later evolved into a starting device.   The prototype

The Antonov Automatic Gearbox

operated by influencing the car's engine and I now realized that this would be an obstacle in introducing the gearbox to the car industry. My new concept was based on a simple three-stepped mechanical automatic gearbox built entirely from parts of the ZF four-speed gearbox used on Peugeot models. With slight modification to some of the parts I now intended to develop a gearbox that would be superior to the hydraulic automatic gearbox produced across the border in Saarbrucken.

I prepared detailed drawings at the mine's engineering office and arranged to meet several of their mechanics to select one to build the prototype. In the workshop in Petite-Rosselle, a tiny village near the border, I met Pierrot Meyer, a short man of forty. He listened quietly to my explanation of the gearbox and then showed me some parts that he had made in his small workshop. The way in which Pierrot talked and handled the parts with his big hands persuaded me that he was the one I should work with. He was an expert with all machine tools and became a good friend of mine; I cannot imagine the success of my gearbox without remembering him. He called our work the big adventure and shared my enthusiasm completely.

Pierrot managed to modify the parts by clever cutting and filing. A few weeks later he assembled the gearbox and we then made a number of tiny modifications until one day we were finally able to assemble the gearbox and prepare the old Peugeot 305 ready to test it. The workshop lacked a hydraulic lift or even a jack. Pierrot lifted the front of the car on to wooden logs and changed the gearboxes by lying under the car.

At first the new gearbox would not function correctly and it turned out that I had installed one of the parts the wrong way round. Patiently and without protest Pierrot took the gearbox apart and reassembled it. The next day I was able to drive the old Peugeot round the workshop yard. My automatic gearbox worked and the car drove surprisingly well.

After testing the prototype, the manager of the Lorraine mines was very impressed. A week later the president of the French national mining concern, Bernard Page, arrived. In an old nearby mine there was a sandy racing track that at places passed dangerously near to the deep pits. I decided to demonstrate the surprising dynamics of my car to Page and took him for a drive on the track. The wheels of the old Peugeot spun because of the high speed, leaving clouds of dust behind us. Passing near the pits I wondered what would happen if the gearbox were to suddenly jam, but this was not the moment to think of adversity. Mr Page seemed truly amazed as he got out of the car.

I drove on and a hundred yards later just in front of the entrance to the workshop the Peugeot came to a sudden halt. Fortunately no-one appeared to notice and I was congratulated by all on my success. On the next day I went to the workshop and saw that Pierrot had already dismantled the gearbox and showed me that many of the parts had drastically overheated because of oil leaks during my wild driving. I studied the abstract sculpture of melted and distorted metal that had once been individual parts and again thought of the many occasions when luck was on my side. If this disaster had happened only a few minutes earlier President Page and I would have ended up in one of the deep pits at the trackside.

The gearbox was quickly repaired and Page personally contacted the president of a French car company to bring my prototype to his attention. As a result of this two of the company's engineers came to Petite-Rosselle to test the performance of the gearbox, arriving in one of their company's latest models fitted with an electronically-operated hydraulic automatic gearbox. This had been recently manufactured and was not yet generally available in production models. One of the engineers had been in charge of its development and I suspected that the intention was to demonstrate the vast gap between my primitive prototype and a modern advanced automatic gearbox for the benefit of my supporters in the mines.

As I sat behind the steering wheel of the seven year-old Peugeot preparing to race against the shiny new car I was unwilling to consider what might happen. It was a sunny day and my friends from the mines were crowding round. I put my foot down hard and noticed after a few yards that I was gaining on the dark red car next to me. As my speedometer indicated 60mph I was well ahead of it with the crowd clapping and cheering. The engineer driving the new car asked me to race him uphill along a road passing by the cemetery of Petite-Rosselle which made a rather steep slope of about half a mile ending at the workshop. At the top of the hill I was twenty yards ahead of the new car fitted with the most advanced automatic gearbox. The long-faced company engineers said that they would arrange to examine my prototype and left in silence.

My investor knew Jean-François Peugeot, a grandchild of the company's founder. The Peugeot family no longer controlled the firm and all Jean-François could do was to arrange a driving test on the test track at Sochaux. A new car would be tested firstly with the standard hydraulic automatic gearbox and then with my prototype automatic in substitution.

Pierrot and I left for Sochaux where he would install my prototype in the new car. Two test drivers took the car on to the track and recorded the results. My prototype was 18.5% more economical with better acceleration and higher maximum speed compared to the standard gearbox. I offered Peugeot the opportunity to reconsider my transmission and returned to Paris a happy man.

Two years after arriving in France it seemed that the door to success had finally opened for me. I had reached my goal by succeeding in building a prototype gearbox better than the existing automatics available. I thought that all I had to do was wait to see what the French car companies would say in the hope that those who had helped me so far would continue to use their influence.

While waiting for the company's decision I decided to return to Bulgaria to meet Mother and my friends. I was curious to see for myself the changes following the fall of the communist regime. It was a beautiful summer and I left by car; a black Peugeot 205 I had bought with the intention of installing a second prototype gearbox in it. I drove through Germany, Austria and Yugoslavia and on the second day parked the car in front of my flat in Sofia. Mother was extremely happy to see me back and I met Rusi and Shego.

There was so much to talk about as I drank coffee at the Shapkite and in the City Garden. It was lovely to see all those familiar places again that had changed so little in my absence. The people in the streets looked the same too and yet there was an obvious change. Everybody was now excited and the nation was deeply divided between communists and democrats. After the opening of the borders Bulgaria appeared even further removed from Western civilization. I drove all the way to the Black Sea and then returned to France taking the same road that I had followed years ago in one of my unsuccessful attempts to defect. I passed through Belgrade, Zagreb

The Antonov Automatic Gearbox

and Ljubljana on my way to Trieste. Late in the afternoon I reached the Sezhana checkpoint where in 1967 I had been arrested. It was now quiet and peaceful and I drove on the deserted road between hills with terraces supported by stone walls. Earlier I had tried to climb those hills in the dark and I wondered what might have happened to me if I had succeeded in my attempt. Having crossed the border I wondered what lay in store for me in Paris.

There was no reply from the French companies. APELOR informed me that the engineers present at the test of my prototype in Petite-Rosselle had reached a negative conclusion. I met some of the engineers and people from the development department of Peugeot but did not get a direct response to my offer until in October both companies turned down the offer to work on my prototype. The situation seemed a complete disaster.

I had offered my prototype only to French car companies. The French government had subsidised my work and APELOR naturally expected me to favour French companies while my friends in the mines urged them to cooperate with me. My investor took the same view and would stand no argument; he was willing to accept total failure of the prototype and the loss of his investment rather than to see the gearbox taken up by foreign companies. If I refused to cooperate I would be left without any financial support.

In France automatic gearboxes were not a particularly important feature. At that time only 2.5% of the cars on the French market were fitted with automatic gearboxes and those mostly in large expensive models. The majority of automatic gearboxes fitted in French cars were imported from Germany while new ones were developed with the cooperation of foreign companies. The French motor industry had enough troubles of its own fighting for survival in an increasingly competitive market and was unwilling to add risk by developing a new automatic gearbox based on an entirely different principle. The people trying my prototype had no influence in the motor industry. Interference at a high level in the corporate structure of these companies was likely to promote even more stubborn resistance by engineers many of whom were reluctant to consider innovations. They would dismiss new inventions with the familiar `no - not invented here'.

Late one night I sat by the window of my little studio with a cup of coffee and a cigarette watching the deserted street. A prostitute stood smoking at the corner of the boulevard. I thought about the twenty years spent attempting to escape from Bulgaria and how I had come to this city and in less than two years succeeded in building the prototype of an automatic gearbox with obvious advantages. Now I had reached a dead end, a refugee without social standing or employment, with large debts and poor spoken French. What could I do with my prototype?

I decided to hold a press conference.

I began by preparing a press kit. Roxanne had returned to the States and I had met Marie-France, an energetic and devoted French woman with a taste for literature. She helped me to edit the text and I borrowed money from the bank, hired a conference room at the Palais de Congrès and sent invitations and a copy of the press kit to a few French newspapers. With my last few francs I bought an expensive suit and a new pair of spectacles. Pierrot came to Paris to help with the presentation of the gearbox.

On 7th September *le Républicain Lorrain* published an editorial entitled *The hardships of a Bulgarian inventor*. There was a photograph of me standing smiling next to the

Peugeot fitted with my automatic gearbox and the editorial explained that despite the advantages of my automatic gearbox I had no chance of promoting it in France and would be forced to seek my luck elsewhere.

I did just that.

A Dutchman, Dan Wysenbeek, was the only person at the press conference who showed interest. He drove the car with the prototype gearbox in Paris and then invited me to Rotterdam to establish a company. I took two copies of *le Républicain Lorrain*, copies of the performance tests of my prototype carried out at Sochaux and my article on theoretical physics and left for Rotterdam with Dan. There we intended to negotiate with potential Dutch investors.

That is how we established a company to promote my automatic gearbox in the car industry. However it took another eight years, a great deal of money and much hard work for Antonov Automotive Technologies to reach its goal.

Chapter Fifteen
Drawing to an End

Together with Dutch investors I founded a company named MAT in 1991 to develop and license the Antonov automatic transmission. This company was not intended to manufacture gearboxes but would sell licences and know-how. The first thing my partners did was to seek other investors while I was charged with building new prototypes of the transmission to be fitted in cars as soon as possible for demonstration to motor manufacturers.

I returned to France to establish a subsidiary company with an office in Paris and a workshop in Lorraine, situated in the small garage in Petite-Rosselle where Pierrot worked.

Within a few months we had installed an advanced and stronger version of the earlier prototype in two Peugeot 205s. These were three-speed transmissions and solid enough to stand abuse from inconsiderate drivers. The prototype cars were faster and more economical than the standard 205 automatic manufactured by Peugeot.

These two cars did an excellent job and once they had been demonstrated we were able to establish a second company, Antonov Automotive Technologies, that attracted new investors able to put up additional resources. In September my partners and I took the prototype cars to the Frankfurt motor show with the intention of establishing new contacts and to demonstrate them to potential licensees. Three major motor manufacturers were interested in the transmission and were prepared to test it. Now seven years later, a prototype commissioned by one of them is being readied for mass production.

Two of Pierrot's sons, Serge and Jean-Claude, came to work at the small garage in Petite-Rosselle. Later we moved the workshop to a larger garage in Diebling, a small nearby town. I frequently commuted between Paris and the workshop in Lorraine; a distance of exactly four hundred kilometres on the beautiful Autoroute de l'Est, crossing serene countryside. During the six years before the workshop moved near to Paris I drove that journey several hundred times by day and night; enjoying the three hours in the car which provided me with an opportunity to peacefully reflect on my work and life.

Excitement always awaited my arrival in Lorraine; I was eager to test again and again the latest gearbox Jean-Claude and Serge had installed in the car - sometimes finishing the job late at night.

In the beginning, the company was badly managed. One of the directors in Rotterdam controlled both operations and finances and seemed determined only to protect his own interests. He was a clever and polished bureaucrat who would interfere with the work and turn everything that had to do with money to his own advantage. He succeeded in structuring the company in such a way that his firm grip on it was perpetuated and he was only interested in selling his shares at the highest possible price. His activities adversely affected the project and my name with it. I therefore contacted the other shareholders and insisted on a reorganisation of the company; threatening to withdraw my services if my demands were refused. There followed a bitter conflict but I pressed on with the reorganisation and won the day. I offered Michael Emmerson, an English accountant, the opportunity to become managing director. Mike accepted the position and soon we reorganised the company. He became my friend and shared with me every step on the long road to launching the Antonov automatic transmission.

To achieve success we only had our prototype cars. During six years we had evolved seven generations of the automatic transmission and installed them in ten different cars. It took fifteen distinct inventions and long hours of improving, researching and testing before my first three-speed transmission evolved into the six-speed automatic that was accepted as the most compact in the world. The race that I began at the hill near the cemetery in Petite-Rosselle never ended; my gearbox simply had to be better than all existing ones in every respect. This was the one and only goal in my work. I would often stand for hours before an engineering drawing or dismantled gearbox wondering how to reach a better result.

However it was not just technical problems with the gearbox that concerned me. I had to deal with everything concerning the wellbeing of the company; its finances, staff, relations with car manufacturers and all aspects of promoting the transmission.

Beside Pierrot, his two sons and Mike, a secretary and engineer joined our Paris office in 1992. By the end of 1997 we had fifteen people on the payroll. It was difficult to find personnel especially at the outset and by employing the wrong people, we suffered. Still, I was successful in assembling a small team to work on the transmission with a degree of efficiency and speed almost unbelievable for a project of that kind; particularly since none of the young people joining me had any prior experience in the motor industry or with vehicle transmissions.

From 1991 promotion became the company's major activity. The transmission was demonstrated to automotive manufacturers at the Paris and Frankfurt shows and the press kept fully informed. I had a major role in these promotional activities; addressing various audiences and press conferences. We toured the world with the prototypes and a series of photographic slides and it was my task to convince the conservative car industry of the advantages of the Antonov transmission.

It was an uphill job. The car industry was not favourably inclined to innovation. I attempted to convince transmission engineers that my automatic gearbox offered many advantages; they all seemed very impressed and agreed with my engineering philosophy but were nevertheless reluctant to become involved. With polite interest, companies worldwide watched every step we took to develop the prototype. We toured Europe, the United States and Japan and it was finally a Japanese company which undertook to investigate the project in 1991 by commissioning us to develop a four-speed prototype for a small city car. The contract was signed in 1992 and the car completed with a four-speed Antonov transmission was ready in 1994 thanks to the Austrian company Steyr-Daimler-Puch of Graz which cooperated with us in its production.

The success of that prototype gave fresh momentum to the company, yet we constantly needed more investment and finding it was anything but easy. Once our Japanese client had become fully involved in developing the transmission, in May 1995 Antonov PLC, registered in Manchester, was quoted on the London (AIM) stock exchange. By that time there were three subsidiary companies in existence in England,

Drawing to an End

Holland and France with me as chairman. In 1997 the company was quoted on the Amsterdam stock exchange too.

Work on developing the gearbox intensified. Once we had fitted electronic control to the four-speed transmission we began work on a six-speed prototype intended to be the most compact automatic transmission in the world. We displayed a scale model of it at the Frankfurt motor show in 1995 while at the Paris show in the following year the prototype car was ready for demonstration.

A contract licensing production of the four-speed automatic was signed with the Indian company Gajra in 1996 with the ultimate intention of installing it in a small Suzuki-designed car manufactured in India. To date that has been the most successful project and this small Indian car equipped with an Antonov transmission was demonstrated at the Frankfurt show in 1997; its qualities finally opening the doors to the world motor industry. At the present time, Antonov Automotive Technologies (AAT) is engaged with eight manufacturers and the total number of projects in hand is greater than our team of engineers.

Still, the sweetest success would be to complete a production prototype for the leading Japanese company that originally undertook to study the project in 1991. Cooperation with its brilliant engineers has provided constant stimulus to the project.

Looking back, I realize that the challenge was far greater than I had imagined. Every single day in the past few years has brought a mass of concerns. Sometimes it seemed to me that the entire enterprise was on the point of collapse. Huge risks had to be taken and results achieved quickly. Some twenty-five million dollars have been successfully invested in the long-term development of the Antonov automatic transmission despite the constant difficulty of raising finance. We felt that it would be even more difficult to convert our labours into an asset with a value in excess of the investment already taken up.

I myself had changed a great deal without noticing it. Although once a lonely and introspective researcher and inventor drinking coffee at the Shapkite in Sofia and generally considered to be a crazy eccentric by my fellow Bulgarians, I was now the president of an international company developing the most advanced transmission technology in the auto industry. My work was not limited to inventions; I was now obliged to be a manager and businessman at the heart of a western capitalist enterprise.

Frankly I did not consider myself to be the most suitable person for this task but was unable to find anyone else better qualified to do the job.

Deep inside me, however, I remained an inventor. In 1991 I began work on my latest four-stroke engine as a leisure activity and Pierrot helped me to build the first prototype. Later in 1995 I founded the Antonov Engine Company and a prototype of the new engine was built and tested at the Technical University of Delft, Holland. Now, second and third developments of this have been evolved and successfully fitted to test vehicles. However, it will take more work and investment yet before my engine can clearly demonstrate its advantages over the classic Otto-cycle engine.

It seems that I made the right choice in 1988 by deciding to develop the automatic gearbox and I am not yet in a position to say whether and when my new engine will be accepted by the car industry.

I found time to continue my hobby as a designer of car bodies and made a full-scale model of a two-seater in the style of the Thirties. Later I bought a small Fiat Topolino of the type produced as the Simca Cinq in pre-war France and restored it to realize a youthful dream.

Yet in fact not one of these demanding activities was my main objective in life.

There was still one other vital task left incomplete and that was to make my fungus research public. In 1991 I realized that success would not come easily or instantly for my automatic transmission. Yet even if it came, it would still be difficult to publish an article about my fungus research in a medical journal; automatic transmissions have very little to do with medicine. I had to find another way to publicise my research.

Then I thought of my earlier passion for literature and the eccentric novel entitled *The Unattainable Calm of a Salesman* that I had written years ago in my tiny attic. In telling his story, my imaginary hero also described the scientific ideas that engrossed him. Perhaps this was a way in which to make public a new theory. The success of my transmission might attract sufficient readers to a story written by me. Perhaps my adventures were worth reading about.

In 1994 I began to write this book with the idea that my story and my successful automatic transmission would be the best way to recommend my fungus research to a wider audience. This was by no means an orthodox way of publicising medical research but it seemed to have merit.

In all the years I have lived abroad I have been aware of the continuing effects of the experiments begun at the end of 1979. During the first two years in Paris I experienced curative crises of the stomach. In the third year, the process of fighting the fungus gradually subsided. I had ceased taking 'M' nine years ago and decided to resume taking it in small doses, being eager to discover whether the process had been completed or if my immune system had lost its capacity to fight the fungus unaided.

After a further two years of taking 'M', in the autumn of 1995 I experienced a series of crises more severe than anything felt before. As Mike and I reached Bombay to negotiate our first licence, I could hardly stand. My blood pressure rose and I became so ill that I panicked at the prospect that I might faint at any moment. I realized once more that the fungus was being discarded from my body as huge quantities of dead tissue peeled from the inside of my mouth at the point where my jaw had been fractured.

During the following day I decided that the crisis was not likely to be repeated and we took the plane to Indore. However, on arrival there I experienced yet another very heavy crisis soon followed by yet more. A series of crises followed during 1996 and became more intensive at the beginning of 1997. The two points where my jaw had been broken in 1961 suddenly became clearly visible and during particularly heavy crises huge amounts of dead tissue peeled off. This process continued for two years although I had abandoned taking 'M' as early as 1995.

The new crises did not differ substantially from those of the 1980s apart from being heavier and more prolonged. They affected the same places - my sinuses, stomach, bowels and my face and skin in general. The huge decomposing heterokaryon of the fungus deep in my body was creating painful crises more persistent than I had expected. At some very agonizing moments I asked myself whether I would survive; it seemed to me that my arteries might clog and cause a loss of consciousness. I did my best to remain awake during the most difficult hours but I knew that no-one could help me and yet the presence of certain people at these times was of great support to me. Diana, a young pretty Dutch girl with blue eyes came to Paris in 1994 to work in the company and she was an ambitious and intelligent girl who shared with me some of my most difficult periods.

Although all that took place confirmed my fungus theory, I concluded that my experiment could not yet be applied as a therapy since the process of fighting the fungus was long, painful and probably dangerous without formal medical supervision.

Drawing to an End

After seventeen years of experiment I still have confidence in my theory of a parasitic symbiosis of the fungus and the human body as described here. I believe that all will turn out well and yet I would certainly not recommend anyone to conduct the experiment in the way that I did before all its effects have been sufficiently evaluated. How far can the process of fighting the fungus continue and how will the human body behave once the parasitic symbiosis has been disrupted?

I cannot answer these questions yet but I hope to be able to do so in the future. Perhaps in years to come medicine will be able to help the sick in a more efficient way and shield future generations from certain diseases.

As I write these lines my story is drawing to an end; at least for the time being. I wish that I had an answer to all the questions that I have wrestled with. One day perhaps I will be able to write a second, more conclusive book but because I am now eager to make my theory and experiment public I am ready to publish the present volume as soon as possible.

Today I live in Paris in the same Boulevard Saint-Germain which I discovered and fell in love with on my second day in the capital. I became a French citizen in Lorraine in 1993. Until my dying day I will love France - this country that has provided me with a home and the opportunity to achieve my ambition - which I was prevented from doing for twenty years.

My son Viktor graduated in the Arts Center in Pasadena, California in 1996 and took a job in Hollywood. At twenty-three he fulfilled the Californian dream that I had when I was his age and sometimes I feel that I can enjoy the shores of the Pacific through his eyes.

On 6th December 1991 my mother died in a Sofia hospital. On the previous day I was at her bedside assuring her that I had finally made it in life. She said that she had always believed in my success. I owe so much to her.

After the fall of Zhivkov's regime the plight of the Bulgarian people worsened. It was not easy to overcome the pernicious influence of communism and this was the case in all East European countries. Yet in Bulgaria the regime was even more rigid and all-pervasive and it would take a long time for the wounds to heal.

I continued to visit my country each year and the pain endured by the people seemed to intensify. Rusi always met me and spent most of his time in my company. Shego and his wife lived in one of Sofia's new housing estates far from the city centre. He still wrote stories for fun. Bobby took a job in Syria.

Once when I walked the streets of Sofia I suddenly felt that I was in a place inhabited by the ghosts of my past. Rusi had just left me and I wondered desperately whom to call. All around me I saw Bulgarians, yet it seemed that the people I once knew had disappeared. After a long walk I decided to return to Paris a day earlier than planned. My new life as an emigré, short as it was, would not allow me to forget the past; perhaps this feeling of isolation and loneliness will accompany me wherever I go.

I am almost fifty-five. Looking back, I realize how dangerous and difficult my life has been. There have been very few moments of real joy and I have known lasting pleasure only in the working of my mind and imagination. I wonder what it was that set me apart from others in the first instance to make my life as it has been? I think that it started perhaps on that very day when my first schoolteacher asked me if I believed in God. I can still visualize the little boy standing by his desk wondering what to say. I am not sure that my life is the best that I could wish for but with all the memories of the hardships I have survived, I know the answer will still be:

Yes, I do.

Paris, January 1998

Chapter Sixteen
Epilogue

This book was originally published in Bulgaria on 27 April 1998. On the occasion of its presentation in Sofia I was suffering from one of the most serious curative crises resulting from the experimentation described in these pages. I had a high fever and barely enough strength to scribble a few words in the first copies of my book for my guests.

At the same time I founded in Sofia the *Antonov Foundation for Medical Research*, the object of which is to organise laboratory experiments in connection with my theory about the parasitic symbiosis of fungi with the human organism and, more specifically, about the role of these fungi in the formation and development of atheromatous plaques. The Foundation began its activities with a modest donation from me.

Following publication, my book soon ranked second in the Bulgarian bestseller list and was out of print within a few weeks. Thanks to publication of the book, I succeeded in bringing together a team of medical experts willing to carry out laboratory experiments on atheromatous plaques. Included in the team were Professor Dr. Gentcho Natchev, a cardiac surgeon at the University Hospital of Sofia and one of the country's leading experts; Dr. Rossen Radev, conducting experimental surgery at the University - the enthusiastic organiser of the team; Dr. Grisha Mateev, a mycologist, and Associate Professor Dr. Todor Kantardjiev, a microbiologist and national consultant on microbiology.

Investigations were carried out with atheromatous plaques from excised arterial sections taken from patients during cardiac surgery at the University Hospital. Under the strictest sterile conditions the arterial tissue was cut across the plaques and then sown on nutrient media for fungi. The experiments were simple and carried out with ordinary standard laboratory materials.

Fungal colonies grew upon most of the sown plaques. Identification of the fungi of these colonies was carried out in Dr. Kantardjiev's laboratory.

Two kinds of fungi had grown upon the plaques in the arterial sections sown on the nutrient media. One of them was the well-known *Rhodotorola rubra*. This fungus is a very rare cause of infections in man and its presence in the atheromatous plaques of blood vessels was a surprise. But the other fungus, about which I had been entertaining suspicions and which in this book I have named *Candida albicans*, proved an even greater surprise. In its growth in the nutrient media it had manifested forms which are inherent in *Candida albicans*, but at the same time fibres had also grown in sizes and forms which had not been described before. *Candida albicans* had hitherto been known to contain fibres 6 to 12 microns thick; but what we saw in the fibres growing on the plaques proved to be up to 20 times thicker than this! These big fibres resembled certain dermatophytic fungi, but unlike them they grew almost only below the surface of the nutrient media, without oxygen. But the most amazing discovery was that they did not manifest any generative cycle at all; the fibres themselves were very slowly growing bigger in the nutrient media.

Was not this a newly-discovered fungal microorganism? Was it a so far unknown form of *Candida albicans*, or was it some other kind of fungus? These questions deserved further and very extensive research, for we still had no clear explanation for them.

All these discoveries made during experiments with atheromatous plaques were more than astounding. As I have mentioned in this book, I had already seen something of these things as early as my first experiments with the decomposition of plaques carried out 18 years ago - for example, much bigger forms of the fungus than those known before. The idea came to me to give some of these fibres, which I had kept since that time, to be investigated in Dr. Kantardjiev's laboratory. Were they the same type, and would they grow again after their long years of isolation between two plastic sheets?

They *did* grow anew and proved to be similar to those on the plaques taken from patients during surgery.

At long last I had succeeded in showing and convincing independent medical men of the existence of these facts. This book, which I wrote to reveal my new medical discoveries, had indeed attained its objective. What now remained to be done was to ensure that the four professionals would be followed in laboratories worldwide by thousands of their colleagues. I told myself that as had been the case hitherto, this might be a difficult task but had to be started at once.

Last April in Sofia I had already promised in a television interview that these medical investigations would be carried out in Bulgaria. On 5th December 1998, the Foundation issued a press announcement there, and I again appeared in a television interview to announce the discovery of the hitherto unknown presence of fungi in atheromatous plaques. I appealed for support for further investigations in Bulgaria and on the following day returned to Paris to continue with my work on the automatic gearbox.

The small team in Sofia carried on with its investigations, but the time had now come for me to find researchers in the developed world. The brief sent to scientists and researchers in the West had aroused interest. The previously unknown strain of fungus is now growing at the University of Paris, and I have registered an intellectual property company in Rotterdam to conduct negotiations with research organisations to develop future therapy.

At the end of April 1999 a second edition of my book was published in Bulgaria with a brief summary of the results of the first experiments there. When I returned to Sofia at that time, I was presented with an exciting surprise; the unknown form of the fungus of last year's experiments, after numerous attempts, had at last propagated and developed a colony on the surface of the nutrient solution!

But as I write today, I am at last sure that my work has borne fruit. This morning, it was confirmed simultaneously in Sofia and Paris that after the closest examination in computer-controlled tests, a totally new microorganism from the human body has been identified, beyond existing understanding and unrelated to any known species. It fills no convenient gap in our knowledge and has no precedent in recent years of scientific discovery.

So now we know what these hitherto unseen fibres growing in the nutrient solution - and most likely in our fellow men in all the nations of the world as well - are. it seems that a happy ending lies ahead for the first English edition of this book and I also hope that it marks the beginning of the universal investigation of the new facts revealed within.

I hope that my labours will now help the many ailing people in this (as it has more than once seemed to me in my life) absurd world. Because, for all that, I believe with all my heart that it is nevertheless still the most wonderful world - and thoroughly worth living in, both in better health and for longer!

Sofia
2 June 1999

Appendix
Bulgaria-The Roots

On my travels round the world in recent years I often came to the realization that the people to whom I talked knew very little about Bulgaria, the country of my birth.

The general understanding of my fatherland as I have seen it through the eyes of various people throughout the world is of a one-time hardline communist country where very little of merit happened. Bulgaria seems to be recognized as a country famous for its top wrestlers and gymnasts, its talented singers and musicians, its beautiful landscape and of course for its yoghurt. The notorious affair of the assassination of the Bulgarian writer Georgi Markov in London by means of a dart fired from an umbrella manipulated by agents of the Bulgarian secret service was perhaps the most widely-known example of my country's resourcefulness in the West.

Because of the general lack of understanding I have summarised the history and spirit of Bulgaria; the small but delightful country where I spent the first forty-four years of my life.

The Cyrillic alphabet used by all Bulgarians in their daily life and by me to write the original edition of my story, marks one of the sublime moments of Bulgarian cultural history. In the ninth century the emerging, dominant Bulgarian State adopted Orthodox Christianity from the fading Byzantine civilization and translated the Holy Bible into a Slavonic language by means of an alphabet specifically devised for that purpose by Cyril and Methodius, two learned brothers who were later canonized. Christianity spread from Bulgaria to other nearby Slavonic states of which Russia and Serbia were the most important.

In later centuries however, the destiny of the Bulgarian people was less illustrious. As the Turks expanded their Islamic empire by conquering vast territories in Southeastern Europe the Bulgarians were forced to remain under Ottoman rule for more than five centuries. During those dark ages most Bulgarians were able to preserve their national identity but at a high cost.

The reason for this is serious and distressing. The Islamic Ottoman Empire did not tolerate any culture or religion other than the true faith. With fanatical barbarity, the Muslims destroyed all remnants of Christianity, crushed resistance and suppressed the remaining infidels.

Isolated in bondage from the surrounding world for ages, the Bulgarian people withdrew into small communities in an attempt to delay the ruthless process of assimilation and cultural substitution practised by their conquerors. This created an introversion resulting in loss of contact with their ancient culture and they were only able to preserve that which could be hidden from Ottoman eyes.

This drama took place during the five centuries of Bulgaria's agonizing isolation and oppression while the remainder of Europe was bathed in the light of the Renaissance, mother of modern civilization. At this time new continents were being discovered and new peoples converted to Christianity, while in miserable isolation in Southeastern Europe the remnants of a once independent nation were held back because of their Christian faith. At the same time that Isaac Newton laid the foundations of experimental science and wrote his commentaries on the Bible, the Bulgarians had lost all written connection with their past and the world in general and were unaware even that the Slavonic translation of the Bible was their creation. In the tiny breathing space allotted to Christianity in Bulgaria by the Ottomans, little of the ancient Slav culture survived.

Christianity survived only because it was perceived as the last bastion of Bulgarian national identity and in a few secluded monasteries and small churches the art of calligraphy and icon painting was tenaciously preserved. It is difficult to imagine what has vanished; spiritual and cultural relics from the past are rare indeed, comprising barely half-a-dozen texts surviving in scattered copies, a few frescoes and abandoned ruins. In Bulgarian legend and song, history is but a myth far removed by time from its factual basis.

For all these reasons, two centuries ago Bulgarian culture and national mentality were quite different from those of other nations on the continent of Europe. The debilitating effort to survive in tiny isolated scattered villages supported by primitive agriculture gave no incentive to invention and creativity nor did it stimulate the adoption of modern civilization. The nation had been able to survive the long period of repression at a high price indeed - at the cost of spiritual exhaustion and backwardness.

The first agitators to awaken the Bulgarian conscience seem of slight intellectual standing in comparison with the intellectual giants of eighteenth century Western Europe. Nevertheless they were faced with the difficult task of arousing a nation sunk into lethargy, virtually illiterate and oblivious of its proud history. For this reason they had to return to the very beginnings.

Paisiy, a monk of the Khilendar monastery, wrote his *A Slav-Bulgarian History* marking the beginning of national revival.

'Oh you ignorant fool, why are you so ashamed to call yourself Bulgarian?' asked Paisiy of his fellow countryman the peasant whose culture could be encompassed by a couple of prayers and a smattering of heathen superstitions. By recounting the story of those ancient times when Bulgaria was illumined by the achievements of its culture and political state, Paisiy was the first to restore its lost self-confidence to this abandoned nation.

After Paisiy, many followed to become Bulgaria's pioneers in the struggle for national enlightenment, to create literature and ecclesiastical independence. Despite its late start the Bulgarian Revival, inspired by advanced Europe, blossomed with limited knowledge and experience but much passion. It was successful too and the Bulgarian Church, education and literature were not only awakened and brought back to life but received official recognition. From its position lagging behind the changing modern world and undermined by revolution in those Ottoman states bordering on Bulgaria, the Turkish Empire could no longer hermetically preserve its Islamic fanaticism and was forced to make concessions to progress.

Christo Botev, a revolutionary and poet, was among the first of the new men of letters in the reborn Bulgarian literature. He was not simply a poet for poetry's sake, for in exile Botev had organised a cadre of rebels with whom he set off for Bulgaria dreaming of instituting a revolt. Botev was killed after his group was routed and quickly defeated after failing to obtain any local support. At the sight of the rebels, the peasants scurried to hide behind the high stone walls of village houses built to shield everything from the outsider's eye.

It is quite possible that the bullet that took Botev's life was from the gun of a fellow rebel since no other argument seemed able to restrain the fanatical courage of the leader who wished to fight to the death a battle already lost. Botev had already chosen death in his poetry if that was to be the price of his dream of a free Bulgarian nation.

Each of the apostles of the Bulgarian Revival dedicated himself to resisting Turkish rule but they all had to fight another more agonizing and draining battle with the darkness clouding the mind of their compatriots. Utopian as they were, the Revivalists knew in their hearts that they stood alone in nurturing dreams of liberty and they formed an insignificant minority dedicated to their cause. The centuries of oppression had left many deep scars in the mentality of the Bulgarian people. *The sword spares a bowed head* says a Bulgarian proverb, expressing the defeatist philosophy of the peasants confined to the patriarchal world of their far-flung villages.

Although initially almost without support, the movement for National Revival soon attracted more and more of the brighter elements of the nation. These exiled dreamers set up governments of fantasy and were often engaged in furious and extended argument in search of the elusive solution to the problem of obtaining their liberty.

The failure of Botev demonstrated that an uprising could only be successful in an environment prepared for it. To establish a network of clandestine committees to kindle the spark of an uprising simultaneously throughout the entire country was a titanic challenge. Yet even more challenging was the need to defeat the might of the Ottoman State with an uprising based on a feeble rebel force.

Vasil Levski was the Bulgarian who took on that daunting task. Disguised and travelling under numerous aliases he criss-crossed the country in all weathers addressing his compatriots with inspiring rhetoric in every village and hamlet. So successful was he that his audience vowed to mount a revolution to gain their liberation.

Firstly Levski had to persuade the Bulgarian people that their uprising would succeed. This required him to overcome half a millennium of ingrained fear in the minds of his compatriots. He succeeded beyond his wildest expectations but was betrayed to the Turks by one of his disciples. Levski was hanged.

What Vasil Levski began was not halted by his death. His ideas for the future attracted more Bulgarians to the flag. This nation that so far was ignorant of its own history and the world around it began to dream of an uprising in every small village, sustained by the dream that the great powers, Russia above all, would support its struggle. This faith in the Slav people of Russia, in *Grandfather Ivan,* was stimulated by the kinship of letters, language, culture and religion and was also inspired by Russia's wars with Turkey.

During the 1870s the world was undergoing profound change. While in Europe the concept of constructing a horseless carriage powered by an internal combustion engine was gaining ground, in a Balkan village a handful of Bulgarians determined to obtain their freedom fashioned a small cannon from the trunk of a cherry tree and prepared to do battle with the Ottoman Empire and its large, well-armed army. The Turkish forces outnumbered the rebels by a vast margin; so what was it that inspired the Bulgarian uprising?

In his *Notes on the Bulgarian uprisings* Zahari Stoyanov gives a vivid account of events. This exceptional man began life as an illiterate shepherd isolated in a typical Bulgarian village and later rose to become a great writer. In one episode Zahari Stoyanov describes how he and a fellow conspirator tried to win over the inhabitants of a small village to the cause of liberation. When his friend's eloquence failed to achieve the desired result Zahari suddenly thought of a trick. He took out a bottle of invisible ink and a pen and demonstrated the working of the mysterious fluid. The effect was overwhelming; bewildered by this magic the peasants readily agreed to join the revolution.

Zahari Stoyanov successfully repeated his trick on many similar occasions.

Having been prepared with so much enthusiasm and thoroughness, the uprising broke out spontaneously in several scattered villages. Georgi Benkovski was quick to seize command and ordered the murder of a few Turks. He knew well that by spilling blood the rebellion would achieve reality and could no longer be ignored. However, this uprising failed to develop on the large scale that had been planned for it and was quickly doomed to fail regardless of the enthusiasm of its protagonists. The consequences were devastating.

The Ottoman authorities drafted regular army forces against the miserably-armed peasants who had undergone no military training. Most terrifying of all were the *Bashibazouks*, irregular Islamic fanatics rushed to crush the revolt.

It is impossible to describe the monstrous cruelty, outrages, arson, massacre, and bloodshed. Even as he watched the burning villages and their terrified inhabitants fleeing for their lives Georgi Benkovski saw the inevitable attainment of his goal despite its continuing invisibility to his defeated fellow countrymen. At his death Benkovski's faith in the revolution was unwavering.

The inevitability of the new order arose from the terror instilled throughout Europe by events in Bulgaria. The massacres of Batak and Peshtera, terrible examples of ruthless retribution against entirely defenceless villages shook the world to its foundations. The Bulgarian revolutionary victory lay in its success in arresting public attention throughout the civilized world. The peasants who believed in their liberation after experiencing the miracle of invisible ink were not betrayed; they were simply unaware that in order to achieve their sacred goal they would have to lay down their lives.

It was only after these events that European public opinion roared its support for the Bulgarian cause and provided Russia with the excuse to declare war on the Ottoman Empire; a conflict that would lead to Bulgaria's liberation.

With Russian victory in 1878 Bulgaria finally gained freedom and independence. Many of the surviving rebels and freedom fighters took part in the war as volunteers and made their ultimate contribution at a vital moment - in the battle of the Shipka Pass in the Balkan mountains. They demonstrated amazing courage in that desperate battle and showed once more that liberty was not easily won.

The early revolutionary visionaries had completed their task. Now it was the time for the founders of the nation, Bulgarians who would now build a new country with boundless enthusiasm despite having little understanding and experience.

The Russians gave the first lessons to their eager pupils who soon learned and demonstrated their ability to continue alone. An independent spirit moved them to take their destiny into their own hands by uniting the country whose territory had earlier been divided and re-shaped by foreign statesmen.

At a new constituent assembly the Bulgarians represented by their most able men laid the foundations of the new state and chose a constitutional parliamentary monarchy. The constitution was modelled on that of Belgium and Ferdinand of Saxe-Coburg Gotha was invited to become Czar after the short initial reign of the Austrian prince Alexander Battenberg.

The new Bulgarian state was founded a century after publication of Paisiy's *History*. But the new generation of Bulgarians no longer wished to dwell in its past. What was

Bulgaria-The Roots

there to look at over one's shoulder? There was much of greater interest ahead within the civilization of Europe. In an overwhelming attempt to annex all the essential elements of civilization simultaneously, the nation rushed headlong into the pursuit of culture, art, science, technology, economics and politics. In its rapturous evolution the nation changed by the day and although the young state was immediately submerged in four wars and was frequently shaken by political turbulence, nothing could hinder its dazzling evolution. Cities and towns were built, industries created, transport installed, universities and theatres established and literature and art flourished.

Ironically Kemal Ataturk, leader of the Reformist Movement that later brought down the decaying Ottoman Empire and introduced the modernisation of Turkey, turned to Bulgaria for inspiration.

Yet in that explosion of energy following centuries of backwardness, a new division took place in Bulgarian society. Many individuals took a great leap forward by rapidly adopting a new culture radically different from that of the sheltered peasant community. More and more Bulgarians adapted to a new way of life and mentality in the thriving towns and cities, creating an ever-widening gap between themselves and their compatriots in the countryside.

Bay Ganyo, a fictional character invented by the author and journalist Aleko Konstantinov now emerged as the embodiment of the feeling of inferiority created by that cultural gap.

Bay Ganyo is the persona of the uncultured person driven by enormous energy and ambition to join Europe but still with the low moral standards of his ancestors. He retains the mentality and the billowing old-fashioned trousers of his fellow villagers despite his comic efforts to conceal his backwardness. Due to inability to adapt himself to his new surroundings, Bay Ganyo creates many awkward and ridiculous situations to which he reacts with unshakeable impudence, vulgar humour and a total lack of sensitivity. The satire of the story has made many Bulgarians share the author's shame thinly disguised behind the irony of his narrative. For Bulgarians Bay Ganyo has become a synonym and the personification of their backwardness.

At the conclusion of World War I, Bulgaria was among the defeated nations. This was the fourth war in a row for a country only forty years old. It was the worst, longest and bloodiest war and brought about national disaster and total annihilation.

The Bulgarians proved to be courageous and dedicated soldiers, but their reward if they survived the conflict was to return to the misery of a ravaged country. Bulgaria's casualties and suffering transformed the national spirit. By evolution towards civilization Bulgaria had joined Europe but this meant little to the downtrodden peasants left with ruined farms.

At this time civilization in general was in a state of crisis. Lenin and his followers seized power in Russia and set out on their journey to change society by bloodshed and terror. Lenin discovered in certain socialist teachings enough arguments to reach the conclusion that only his philosophy was correct and that dissent had to be crushed by violence. Moreover as it became obvious that nothing was sacrosanct including religion (an opium to the people, in his view) it became obvious that he was preparing for world revolution after the conversion of Mother Russia to his faith.

Among the suffering hungry masses in Russia there were plenty of people ready to take up arms to follow Lenin, as they would rather believe his promises than be exploited by the capitalists. In the same way the politics of revolution appealed to sections of the Bulgarian populace, too.

With a common language and culture it was not so strange that some Bulgarians were won to the cause of world revolution. Lenin himself took notice of that fact and wrote somewhere in his chaotic notes of his intention to learn Bulgarian. Yet because of his preoccupation with the liquidation of as many priests as possible he noted elsewhere that he was running out of time to accomplish this resolve. Nevertheless his Bulgarian followers very well understood his intentions despite his use of the Russian language, and proceeded to organise bloodbaths at home in what became a failed attempt to seize power.

During that difficult time Boris III was crowned Czar of Bulgaria following the abdication of his father Ferdinand. Boris's reign began with his miraculous survival of two attempted assassinations. The first attempt by bullet, missed the Czar by a mere couple of inches in an ambush in one of the Balkan passes. On the second occasion a huge bomb concealed by communists in the church of St Cyriaca in Sofia exploded only a few seconds before his arrival, killing many hundreds. To be a good Czar under such circumstances was a challenge indeed.

Czar Boris III showed remarkable talent in his determination to create a democratic state in such an intolerant political climate. Remarkably, he succeeded and the time came when Bulgaria was able in turn to teach a lesson to many of its former mentors who now found themselves afflicted by outrage and political troubles too.

Under Czar Boris III the country experienced a short period of national prosperity. Bulgarians became affluent; the economy and trade were booming, initiative was given opportunity and European civilization entered into everyday life, inspiring the national culture and spirit to aspire to reach world standards of achievement.

Naturally enough progress was concentrated on Sofia, Bulgaria's largest city and the source of the nation's prosperity. At the beginning of the twentieth century it was hardly more than a large village, yet forty years later Sofia had profoundly changed to become one of the most charming modern cities on the continent. Beautiful houses, streets and entire quarters sprung up in the enchanting atmosphere of this proud and flourishing period of industrially-based civilization.

However, the gap between those driven by aspiration towards the highest human achievements and those who never removed their old-fashioned full-bottomed baggy breeches posed a problem more acute than ever before. Hardly sixty years had passed from the time when a small cherry tree cannon had represented the peak of Bulgarian technology to the dazzling aeroplanes designed and produced by the new generation of Bulgarian technicians. This immense gap in achievement between individuals was a new experience for the nation. The jealous, subconscious hatred of those backward members of the community towards their progressive rivals formed the emotional basis of communism in a way which endured and increased in power with disastrous results.

After the initial German successes at the beginning of the Second World War which abruptly brought to an end the romantic decade of the Thirties, Mussolini, anxious to avoid eclipse by his Teutonic fellow fascists from Berlin, decided to invade Greece. Hitler was appalled by this totally unannounced act of folly which clashed with preparations for his own invasion of Russia, despite the 1939 secret non-aggression pact. The Greek army, able to muster only a single serviceable tank, somehow managed to halt the Italian advance and Mussolini's troops were driven into ignominious retreat. Against his will, Hitler was forced to draft the Wehrmacht to Greece to end this emergency, followed by an immediate about-turn back to the icy steppes of the Soviet Union. This adventure had a decisive effect on the role of Bulgaria in the war.

Bulgaria-The Roots

Unnerved by Mussolini's action, Hitler ordered the three Balkan countries Bulgaria, Yugoslavia and Rumania to create an alliance and grant the German army free passage to Greece. Aware of the likely consequences, the political leaders of the three countries signed the treaty without dissent. Only the Serbs brought down their government and rejected the treaty; preferring the atrocities of war.

Boris III rejected the option of opposing Hitler but reduced the degree of collaboration with Germany to a record low - not a single Bulgarian soldier fought in the war and not a single Bulgarian Jew was deported. This very possibly cost him his life since after refusing again to defer to Hitler at a meeting in 1943, Boris III is believed to have been poisoned. The beloved Czar died a couple of days after his return to Sofia, plunging the country into deep mourning.

The Czar's old communist enemies had already begun their armed struggle against the State and as I return to the subject of communism I realize how difficult it is to explain events with the use of conventional concepts; the norms of humanity having been so heavily distorted.

During the last decades of the nineteenth century, European public opinion reacted strongly to the Ottoman atrocities in putting down the Bulgarian Revolt and Russia was subsequently persuaded to challenge Turkey to a war which led to Bulgaria's eventual liberation. However in order to achieve that success the public had to know what was going on and even at the dawn of the telegraphic era Europe knew what was happening in remote Bulgarian villages within the antiquated Turkish Empire.

Something very extraordinary and deep-seated must have taken place after World War I if it now became possible for millions of people to be tortured, murdered or exiled by services of the state specially created for that purpose without general knowledge despite the more advanced means of communication now available. Moreover inhuman monsters such as Lenin who personally gave instructions that no killings were to be recorded, were hailed as messiahs of the new order by their intellectual supporters in the civilized world. Lenin however only laid the foundations of this repressive society. As the regime took a more monstrous form under Stalin even the fragments of information about repression that had occasionally reached the public vanished forever. Instead communism now gained in stature and engaged the imagination of many people throughout the world; it is truly amazing how leading intellectuals believed in this demented demagogy. It was quite acceptable to ridicule Hitler as Chaplin did in *The Great Dictator* but to attempt to mock Stalin was frankly inappropriate.

Behind the facade erected before the world by communism Stalin established his paranoid dictatorship on a scale and degree of cruelty, mass murder and torture surpassing all human imagination. Stalin created a theory of the intensification of the class struggle to justify these killings; other scientific aspirations urged him for example to hold forth on the subject of linguistics. But Stalin's major contribution was his system of repression which continued relentlessly in an atmosphere of perpetual self-glorification and applause. Surrounded by vast portraits and sycophants, he proceeded to destroy the greatest number of his fellow countrymen of any dictator in history, leaving a model of ultra-efficient perpetual dictatorship to his earnest disciples Mao, Castro and the others.

In this cruel farce staged to create a pleasant and *progressive* image of the communist nightmare there was a role for the Bulgarian Georgi Dimitrov.

Following Lenin's instructions, Dimitrov had organised bloody revolution in Bulgaria during the 1920s. When this was suppressed he fled to Soviet Russia by boat and ten years later emerged in Berlin where he was immediately arrested and accused of setting fire to the Reichstag. Despite a vociferous campaign against the communists the Nazi leaders failed to prove to the German court that Dimitrov and his associates were guilty.

This was acclaimed by the communists who declared Dimitrov a hero and victor over Nazism. Amid bombastic propaganda and spectacular displays for the benefit of the world communist movement Stalin rescued Dimitrov and his comrades. Instead of following through with a vigorous world revolution Stalin created the *Comintern* and appointed the servile Dimitrov, now a distinguished international figure, to be its general secretary.

This was for the sake of appearances and just like Stalin's other creations the reality was a nightmare. By means of murder and repression among his closest circle Stalin reduced the survivors to a state of abject fear and inertia, turning them into pathetic puppets and lickspittles. The higher their standing in the system the more terrified they were to incur the tyrant's wrath. Stalin sent President Kalinin's wife to a labour camp and the president promptly shut up. He took to slapping some of these distinguished leaders in the face and they seemed to accept this as normal, frightened that they too might be incarcerated. In this system the Comintern was no exception and treated international leaders exactly like their Soviet colleagues. Dimitrov was quick to learn; his two Bulgarian associates were sentenced and died in a camp after their comrade in accordance with the convention testified against them in the people's court.

Dimitrov himself grew a moustache and took to smoking a pipe like Stalin; complying exactly with all accepted dogma whenever he made an announcement. Having reached the necessary high degree of unquestioning submission he was appointed leader of the Bulgarian communist movement in Moscow.

Some of the Bulgarian communists held Utopian ideas about the movement, the Soviet Union and Stalin himself. Some of them were idealists and fanatically and freely took part in conspiracies since they accepted at face value all the fantastic fables about the proletariat and the bourgeoisie. Others among this great variety of people were just simple uneducated types seeking comfort for their confused minds in communism.

The leadership itself however was in the hands of the uncompromising lackeys at the Moscow Centre who simply passed on orders. Stalin had the clear objective of annexing Eastern Europe and while bargaining with Churchill and Roosevelt at Yalta had already specified those countries in which his work on linguistics was to be welcomed.

At this point in my story I would like to change the course of history and find myself in a country where there would be no murder and repression. Unfortunately I have no option but to accept that I was born at the beginning of 1944 in Sofia and the ridiculous linking of all these circumstances and events of which I have given a somewhat subjective account would of necessity determine my whole life.

At that time the alliance of Bulgaria with Germany had dragged the country into war with the United States and as a result Sofia was regularly bombed by Flying Fortresses. At the beginning of the autumn of 1944 the advancing Russian army was approaching the Bulgarian frontier and few among the Bulgarian populace were prepared to make sacrifices for their German allies. Caught between the opposing bombardments from the German military occupation and the approaching Russian army, many Bulgarians felt utterly insecure and could not imagine a future.

Bulgaria-The Roots

The Bulgarian government, feverishly seeking any way in which it could join forces with the West, arrested and disarmed the German military units within its territory. The Soviet Ambassador in Sofia was offered all possible facilities for the Soviet army and the government proposed immediate military action in the war against Germany.

In return Stalin declared war on Bulgaria despite the country having resisted Hitler's coercion and despite the fact that it had maintained neutrality throughout the most difficult part of the war when the Russians were in retreat. The communist resistance forces were instructed to take over power on the same day that the Soviet army entered the country. There was no resistance - in fact quite the opposite - for the partisans and Russian forces were welcomed with open arms.

The armed communist movement in the country had increased in number as the Soviet troops approached. As always the stronger party seemed most attractive.

The vicious image of Fascism causing untold death and misery to millions served Stalin well as justification to hunt down and punish the fascists; an ideal point of departure for the establishment of a machine of repression. The old police forces were liquidated and replaced by a *people's militia* formed of communist partisans; similarly a *people's court* replaced the established judiciary. But behind all these anonymous manifestations of the *people* stood the menacing Dimitrov and his circle, well-drilled in repressive dictatorship by Moscow. As for the people - there were sufficient Bay Ganyos ready to pick up a stick and thrash around them without mercy. Many of those sentenced by the people's courts were clubbed to death; sentence often being pronounced after the execution had taken place.

A flood of repression swept across the entire country and the murder of people who had been declared fascists for a wide range of reasons whether personal or not - sometimes with no reason at all but because of the general hatred of the backward element of the population for the progressives - exceeded the number of communists killed in the resistance. The new victims were given no chance to put up any opposition but were simply caught and beaten to death.

It was still again a *people's* court that pronounced the members of the National Assembly, all former ministers and Prince Cyril, brother of the Czar, guilty and then sentenced them to death. All of them, more than three hundred, were summarily executed. Milling around the Court of Justice `the people' shouted `death!' when asked for their advice by loudspeaker.

Ten thousand citizens or more were killed as `enemies of the people' in a manner more excessive than the Ottoman massacres before the foundation of the Bulgarian State and thousands more were sent to languish in prison or concentration camps. The repressive machine of the bloodstained executioners laid the foundations of communism and most of these hangmen established successful careers in the world of merciless repression. `We have taken this power with blood and will only surrender it with blood' some of them would say later after having spent the greater part of their life enjoying privileges reserved exclusively for the Establishment.

Beside the repression, Bulgaria suffered great human loss as a result of sending the army in the final stage of the war against the Germans. But this was only a beginning and well-instructed in Stalin's methods, Georgi Dimitrov returned to Bulgaria to apply personally all that he had learned to destroy Bulgarian democracy and replace it with a Stalinist dictatorship supported by new repression and demagogy.

A couple of years later Georgi Dimitrov became *the leader* of a decimated Bulgaria that under his direction would cheer on *the great leader and teacher of all peoples* Joseph

Vissarionovich Stalin. In order to realize this aim, all political opponents were massacred and their parties banned; the monarchy and the constitution itself were destroyed and in its place a *people's* republic and a *people's* democracy proclaimed. Private ownership of capital and property was abolished. The country's borders were closed, camps established everywhere, arrest and torture for sins of imperialism and bourgeoisie applied to ever-increasing numbers of people based on a class system of distinction. Purges and exiles became commonplace and copious files were maintained on all citizens. Having been resurrected after centuries of darkness, Bulgarian civilization, culture and democracy were again mercilessly crushed by Stalin's primitive henchmen so that yet another country could proclaim his greatness. As everywhere else communism drew its basic energy from the hatred of the backward for the progressive and in Bulgaria this hatred had been boiling up for centuries. The nation lost its best and most progressive citizens so that Bay Ganyo could come to power. As for Dimitrov; beside organising the murders and repressions he achieved distinction by his polished phraseology and his manifest hatred for the intelligent. His habit of offering his opinion without hesitation and in total ignorance on all subjects probably cost him his life however.

After the war Stalin's paranoia and megalomania increased. Tito, another trainee of the Comintern, applied the master's lessons in order to establish his dictatorship in Yugoslavia. However he did it for his own sake and refused to submit to the will of his master. That infuriated the tyrannical Stalin and he began to suspect the subservient Dimitrov too, since the latter had been foolish enough to declare interest in forming a federation with Yugoslavia.

Dimitrov was called back to Moscow for medical treatment and died shortly afterwards. Stalin gave orders for the mummification of his body and the Bulgarians had the honour of acquiring the first mausoleum in modern times after Lenin's great original. Now they could bow and march before this structure in honour of other tiny tyrants during the forty years before communism would finally collapse leaving the country impoverished, devastated, backward and isolated from Europe and the rest of the world. At that point the crowd spontaneously converted the mausoleum into a public lavatory.

These are the events that mark the period and the setting of my story.

Index

Academy of Fine Arts, 51, 52, 57, 63
Adriana, 19-21
Anne, 140
Anton (father), 13, 14, 17, 18, 20, 25, 44, 81
Antonov Automotive Technologies (AAT), 155, 157
Antonov Engine Company, 157
Antonov Foundation for Medical Research, 161
Antonov PLC, 156
ANVAR, 148
APELOR, 149, 150, 153
Applied Design Centre, 53
Atheromatous plaques, 104, 107, 109, 162
Avramov, Michail, 145, 146

Bandaratsite (pop group), 52
Benkovski, Georgi, 166
BMW, 99, 100, 118
BMW 315 car, 16
Bobby (Boris Staykov), 23-25, 28, 30, 47, 49, 50, 57, 64, 69, 100
Boris III, Czar, 168, 169
Borislava (grandmother), 13
Botev, Christo, 164
Branimir, 29, 30, 64, 80, 81
Brezhnev, 53, 59, 73, 110, 134
Burkart, 146, 147, 149

Candida Albicans, 103-114, 161
Castro, Fidel, 41
Centre of Industrial Aesthetics, 73, 74
Chernenko, 138
Cholakov, Stoyan, 98, 99, 118
Christov, Christo, 66
City Garden, 19, 26, 28
Comsomol (Communist Youth Organisation), 24, 26, 33, 37

Darwin, 50
Diana, 158
Diesel, Rudolf, 77
Dimitrov, Georgi, 169-172
Dolni Lozen, 11, 26
Douglas (uncle) 15, 16

Edith (wife), 142, 146, 147
Einstein, 50
Embassy, British, 113
Embassy, United States, 113
Embassy, West Germany, 113, 118
Emmerson, Michael, 156, 158
Evgeni (brother), 15, 16
Evgenia (mother) 11-14, 18, 31, 42, 152
Evgeniev (Ministry of Interior), 84, 85

Feynman (*Lectures on Physics*), 62
Fiat *Topolino*, 32, 157
Ford 12M, 51
Four-stroke engine (Antonov), 77-84, 87, 90, 92, 95, 120, 121, 139, 157
Frankfurter Allgemeine, 130

Gajra, 157
Galya, 71, 72, 74, 75, 80, 82
Ganyo, Bay, 167
Gaydarov, Georgi, 85-87, 89-91, 93, 107, 115
Gearbox, Antonov automatic, 48, 145-154
Genscher, Hans-Dietrich, 116, 119-121, 127, 129, 135, 137, 139, 147
Georgiev, Zdravko, 73
Germanov, Milcho, 122, 123
Gorbachev, 139, 140

Hasek, Jaroslav (*The Good Soldier Svejk*), 29
Hegel, 50
Helsinki Agreement, 73, 116, 129
Hitler, 14, 169
Hungarian Revolution, 27, 28

Institute for Inventions, 84, 88

Kaprelyan, Prof., 130-133, 139, 147, 149
Kardzhali, 39-45
Kennedy, John F, 40, 41
Konstantinov, Aleko, 167
Kotsev, Inspector Lyubomir, 120, 128
Kruschev, 35, 36, 41, 53, 54

Larisa, 141
Lasch, Prof. Hans Gotthard, 130, 131, 134, 139, 140, 149
L'Automobile, 70
Lenin Higher Mechanical and Electrotechnical Institute, 47
Lenin, 41, 82, 89, 168
Levski, Vasil, 165
Lyuben (brother), 14
`Lyubo', 88, 90, 91, 93, 102, 108, 140

'M' (anti-fungal antibiotic), 103-116, 124, 125, 128, 133-135, 137, 140, 158
Malo Buchino, 14
Mariana, 28, 57
Marie-France, 153
Marion, 90
Markov, Georgi, 54, 163
MAT, 155
Max Planck Institute, 117, 118, 134, 139, 147, 149
Meccano, 20
Mercedes-Benz, 99
Merlebach (Lorraine), 150
Meyer, Pierrot, 151, 152, 156
Milev, Dimitar, 52
`Mitko', 47, 48, 50, 58, 64
Mitterrand, 116, 148
Mladenov, 121, 127, 129, 147
Montand, Yves, 31
Mussolini, 168, 169

Nakov, Volodya, 116
Nikolov, Alexander, 63
Nikolov, Nikolay, 78, 80, 81, 86, 89
Nikolov, Professor, 130-132
Nomenclatura, 68, 95

Oswald, Lee Harvey, 41
Otto (grandfather), 13
Otto, Niklaus, 77

Paisiy, 164
Petite-Rosselle, 151, 152, 155
Petkov, Petko, 71
Peugeot, Jean-François, 152
Physics, thesis etc., 65, 96
Piaf, Edith, 31
Polikarov, Prof. Azarya, 66
Popov, Dr. Nikola, 116
Povest ob Avtomobyle (Story of the Car), 27
Prague Spring, 59
Progress Centre, 95, 96, 98
Protogerov, Slavcho, l06, 107, 110, 112, 122, 128, 130

Quattroruote, 70

Renault 8 car, 64 69, 79
Renault 16 TS car, 64, 66, 69
Républicain Lorrain, 153, 154
Rhodotorola rubra, 161
Rosalina, 19, 20
Rositsa, 52, 60-64, 68, 69, 70, 74, 79

Roxanne, 147, 149, 153
Rubenbauer, Lothar, 99
Rusi, 52, 57, 139, 159

Sergey, 111, 112, 115, 116, 119, 121, 123
Shapkite Café, 59, 106, 112, 157
Shego (Georgi Georgiev), 26, 30, 47, 57, 100, 111, 118, 125, 129
Shopps, 11
`Slavcho', 11, 15, 18, 21
Slavkov, 71
Sokolov (racing driver), 16
Stalin, 169, 170, 172
State Security, 34, 35, 43, 54, 55, 63, 75, 76, 78, 85, 87, 89, 91, 93, 98, 102, 112, 115, 120, 127, 134, 137
Steyr-Daimler-Puch, 156
Stoena (grandmother), 11-15, 17, 18, 23, 25, 31, 42, 49, 53, 58, 63, 68, 99, 133
Stoyanov, Zahari, 165
Strigachev, Prof., 66
Süddeutsche Zeitung, 129, 130

Tanya (aunt), 15, 16, 27, 35
Tarev, Inspector, 34, 35
Technica Foreign Trade Society, 96-98, 102
Terziev, Bogomil, 74, 75, 78
Teske, Rudolf, 114-119, 123, 133, 149
Tosho (Todor Tolev), 88-91, 100, 106, 110, 117
Tsvete, l00, 111, 122, 125-127, 129, 130

Udrev, Vladi (uncle) 19-21
Uzunov, Col. Christozko, 86, 91, 93, 98, 101, 102, 107, 108, 110, 112, 122, 123, 128, 140

Vanga (clairvoyant), 110, 141, 142
Vera, 49
Victoria (fortune-teller), 58
Viktor (son), 65, 78, 110, 130, 133, 135, 146, 148, 149, 159
Violet (sister), 25, 30
Volvo, 99

Wankel, Felix, 28
Wankel engine, 64, 92, 97
Wysenbeek, Dan, 154

Yakimov, Yakim, 67, 71
Yankov, Yanko, 116
Yugoslavia, 55, 75

Zagreb, 60, 61
Zhivkov, 53, 89, 101, 112, 115, 117, 138, 159
Zhivkova, Ludmilla, 122